with specific tools designed to find calm and peace in the maelstrom. Thus armed, the practitioner is better able to repair the world, heal relationships, and raise the next generation. I can see myself referring to it frequently. It will be a terrific resource.
Sharon Dickinson, MDiv, Coordinator of Reiki, Brigham and Women's Hospital, Boston, MA

Elise Brenner and Nancy Spatz offer readers a wealth of mind-body practices based in Reiki teachings. The very relatable real life anecdotes contained throughout the book demonstrate how simply and quickly these tools can be used to shift perspective when faced with challenging situations that arise in daily life. Through self-Reiki practice we can become more resilient, more compassionate, and more peaceful beings. As a bookstore owner, I look forward to sharing their work with people seeking to develop these qualities in themselves.
Cathy Kneeland, Owner, Circles of Wisdom bookshop, Methuen, MA

What a great gift Elise Brenner and Nancy Spatz have given us in this beautifully crafted book designed for embracing the self-care practices contained within the system of Reiki. From the opening paragraph's clear and concise description of Reiki, to the detailed and carefully researched evidence behind the mechanisms of this gentle healing practice, readers will be able to easily understand and embrace the traditional Japanese Reiki methods of cultivating inner peace and self-compassion. The authors gently and meticulously guide us through each of these practices and then use anecdotes and reflections to help deepen our awareness. Every question you have ever had about Reiki as a self-care practice is answered in this gem of a book, including population-specific challenges and how deepening our own practice can help ease social suffering. This is a must-read for Reiki practitioners as well as those who have a desire to deepen their understanding of the meditative and self-healing practices of Reiki. This book is life-changing. It will definitely be on my required reading list for all of my students.

Helene Williams, BSN, RN, Reiki in Health Care Consultant

When I was a harried pre-med undergraduate taking a course called "the Sociology of Medicine" a cardiologist from the Beth Israel Hospital came to give a lecture. It wasn't about the diseases of heart and blood vessels (at least not directly), but rather Dr. Herb Benson taught us about the Relaxation Response – simply put, how breathing and meditation could promote equanimity and calm. It worked – at least it helped me get through my organic chemistry test. A few years later in medical school I learned about how I could actually slow my heart rate and blood pressure with similar techniques that also employed biofeedback.

Fast forward to my current work as a leukemia specialist at a major academic center. Not to mention the chaos of a busy family, professional stresses such as promotion issues, research funding shortfalls, and overwork abound. But of course such matters pale in comparison to the physical and emotional burdens faced by my patients for whom serious illness coupled with painful and exhausting medical procedures are the norm. I have seen enormous individual strength marshalled.

External help in these struggles is always needed. Help can be provided by families and by medical professionals such as social workers, psychologists and psychiatrists. But what about techniques taught by expert practitioners that patients can use to summon inner strength and peace in the midst of their worlds being on fire? Brenner and Spatz write eloquently about the path to spiritual well-being made possible by self-Reiki practice. This beautiful strategy is a key tool in our medical shed to help patients – and for that matter, all of us – negotiate the inevitable lumps and bumps – and mountains – that happen during life.

I find it so inspiring that out of tribulation can come beauty, that a better path can be found even in darkness, and that peace can be found even in the worst of times. There is a clear physiological basis to Reiki – which I as a scientist certainly appreciate. But it is likely more than ironic that from the beginning of my career with Benson, and through its latter stages with Brenner and Spatz, I was introduced and reintroduced to mindfulness. Whether singled out as such or not, it was and will be critical to living and helping well.

Richard M. Stone, MD, Director, Adult Acute Leukemia Program at Dana-Farber Cancer Institute, and Board member of the Medical Oncology Board of the American Board of Internal Medicine

Scholarly, thought-provoking, and filled with clinical acumen, Brenner and Spatz have composed a comprehensive guide to the nature and practice of Reiki at a time when it is most welcome in our world as we live through current turbulence, including the pandemic of 2019-21. This lively and lovely text offers children, adolescents and adults alike readily accessible practices to steady the mind and restore well-being. Brenner and Spatz are grounded in an understanding of child, adolescent and adult development, and they have modified Reiki practice to meet the needs of individuals of all ages. Parents will find it heartwarming to practice Reiki with their children and share with them the calming space where more authentic relationships can blossom. This book is clearly a gem and a welcomed resource for clinicians and the persons in their care!

Rosemarie E. Camoscio, MD, Child, Adolescent, Adult Psychiatrist

Reiki: A Self-Practice To Live in Peace with Self and Others has arrived at an unprecedented time of individual and societal stress over the pandemic and social unrest. Drs. Brenner and Spatz have successfully presented a concise historical review of the origins of Reiki as well as the basis for the healing effects of Reiki on the mind, body, and spirit. The emphasis on *hara* breathing in conjunction with hands-on healing and meditation techniques offers clear and practical instruction to achieve individual inner peace and calm and share this empowerment with others. The authors have skillfully outlined Reiki techniques for the individual to develop a sense of inner strength to meet life's challenges, and through the teachings of the 5 Precepts develop a connection with and compassion for others. This book offers an excellent resource for those of us in healthcare to employ in our personal lives, and I also look forward to sharing this great contribution with colleagues and patients.

Nancy Efferson-Bonachea, MD, Ophthalmologist, Vitreo-retinal Specialist Private Practice since 1996, Tufts Medical School MD 1990, Washington Hospital Center Internship Internal Medicine 1990-1991, Ophthalmology Residency and Vitreo-retinal fellowship at Georgetown University Medical Center

The ultimate guide to self-healing the soul, interpersonal relations and the world, *Reiki: A Self-Practice To Live in Peace with Self and Others* provides the reader a captivating and practical guide for developing a strong self-Reiki practice. This book could not be more timely in light of current affairs as our nation reels from a pandemic and highly escalated racial tensions. Brenner and Spatz have hit a homerun for energy healing with this guide that provides real-world examples making it easy to understand how Reiki assists in healing. A must-read!

Maisie Raftery, Publisher, *Natural Awakenings* magazine, Boston

Thank you for this book. Such a valuable resource for these times personally and collectively. I feel supported, guided and comforted simply by reading it.

Lonnie Poland, President, Vermont Reiki Association, Physical

Therapist, Certified Yoga Teacher, Reiki Teacher/Practitioner, and Mindfulness Facilitator

What a joy to find a resource that reminds me that self-care is not a luxury but an integral part of the Reiki journey. Drs. Brenner and Spatz create a path through the confusion and upheaval of today's times to an oasis of centered calm and clear thinking. The principles contained in this book allow the reader to integrate beloved basics with a broader perspective of Reiki self-care that leads to a more loving practice. I know that this will be a reference that I will use often.

Barbara Gray, Master Reiki Practitioner

This book is a wonderful resource for anyone who wants to learn about Reiki. Mind-body practice has so much to offer us, especially during difficult times.

Valerie Leiter, PhD, Professor of Public Health & Sociology, Chair, Department of Public Health Simmons University; author, *Their Time Has Come: Youth with Disabilities on the Cusp of Adulthood*; editor, *The Sociology of Health and Illness*

Reiki: A Self-Practice To Live in Peace with Self and Others

Reiki: A Self-Practice To Live in Peace with Self and Others

Elise Brenner, PhD
& Nancy Spatz, MD

BOOKS

Winchester, UK
Washington, USA

JOHN HUNT PUBLISHING

First published by O-Books, 2021
O-Books is an imprint of John Hunt Publishing Ltd., 3 East St., Alresford,
Hampshire SO24 9EE, UK
office@jhpbooks.com
www.johnhuntpublishing.com
www.o-books.com

For distributor details and how to order please visit the 'Ordering' section on our website.

ISBN: 978 1 78904 709 7
978 1 78904 710 3 (ebook)
Library of Congress Control Number: 2020942459

A CIP catalogue record for this book is available from the British Library.

Design: Stuart Davies

UK: Printed and bound by CPI Group (UK) Ltd, Croydon, CR0 4YY
Printed in North America by CPI GPS partners

We operate a distinctive and ethical publishing philosophy in
all areas of our business, from our global network of authors to
production and worldwide distribution.

Contents

Disclaimer

This book is not intended to be a substitute for professional medical advice, diagnosis, or treatment. Always seek the advice of your physician or other qualified health provider with any questions you may have regarding a medical condition. Never disregard professional medical advice or delay in seeking it because of something you have read in this book.

This book is dedicated to two dads, Leon Brenner, PhD and Edward Spatz, MD, who taught their daughters, Elise Brenner and Nancy Spatz, about unconditional love and how to cross bridges. A lifelong teaching that both our dads shared was to be grateful and appreciative for every good moment because living our lives is not easy or predictable.

book, I have used techniques described to help an eight-year-old boy whose foster mom brought him in because he was so scared he was going to die from coronavirus that he was not able to eat or do any of his normal activities. An adolescent boy with ADHD who was having insomnia and behavior difficulties will be helped by the practice of *hara* breathing and practicing the Pause when he interacts with his brother or other kids in school. *Gassho* meditation was shown to a teenage girl struggling with obesity, depression and anxiety.

As a co-owner of a large pediatric practice, we have seen that workplace stress and burnout are real. Part of that stress comes from people bringing in stress from their own lives, balancing the busyness of work and family life, as well as the demands that work brings and the variety of personal interactions that it necessitates. As a leader, it is crucial to be able to help our staff; Reiki self-practice is something we can teach to our staff and help them so that they are free from anxiety and fear, which may prevent them from reacting adversely to patient or coworker needs, and become more open to be able to provide compassion to our patients.

In addition, as a busy professional, juggling demands of family, patients, staff, as well as trying to help the children of the community and state, self-Reiki practice is a centering technique which can help us realize we can coexist with anxiety and worry but that it does not have to define us. We can, with the different techniques, stay true to ourselves, and be more effective with our goals of helping others, with compassion and love and joy, even when the emotional and physical demands of our jobs and lives are potentially all consuming.

Reiki: A Self-Practice To Live in Peace with Self and Others, and its universal precepts of not fueling anger, worry, living honestly, with gratitude and compassion, shows us ways that we can coexist with differences, being kind and true to ourselves and to our fellow humans. It shows us ways we can heal and love ourselves as well as others. Especially in these days where distancing is becoming the norm, it shows us more ways we can connect. It is a refreshing antidote to the loneliness and pain that has swept our nation even with the immediacy of personal interaction that social media provides.

Our hope is that word spreads of this amazing healing book and practice.

Elizabeth Homans McKenna, MD, FAAP is co-owner of and pediatrician at Healing Hearts Pediatrics, PLC, with multiple offices in metropolitan Phoenix, Arizona. She is a graduate of Boston University School of Medicine in 1989. She was trained as a pediatrician during her residency at the University of California, San Francisco Medical Center from 1989-1992. She is active in child advocacy and access to care issues in Arizona. She is recipient of the American Academy of Pediatrics Special Achievement Award and the Kevin Keogh Community Award in 2016. She has a wonderful husband and three children, and one grandchild, and enjoys spending time with her family and friends, riding her horse, and walking her dogs.

Introduction: Welcome to the Possibilities

We welcome you here to discover the possibilities that self-Reiki practice has to offer. Whether you are new to Reiki or not, let's start with a helpful definition: Reiki is a mind-body-spirit healing and meditation practice from Japan that promotes health and well-being, mindfulness, resilience, and aliveness. All of us can draw on Reiki mind-body skills to claim our strengths, sustain our well-being day-to-day, and address challenges, both big and small, personal and societal. The self-practice of Reiki is an integrative mind-body-spirit approach that is accessible to people of all ages, backgrounds, and health conditions.

In our hearts, we all want to live *on* purpose and *with* purpose. The teachings and practices of self-Reiki give us an essential resource we can incorporate into our everyday lives to bring in, reach for, and claim our inner qualities and awareness so that we can live intentionally. By living intentionally, we invite physical, emotional, and spiritual well-being. You will learn how self-Reiki practice brings a sense of balance, aliveness, and peacefulness into everyday moments, as well as into moments when we feel physically and emotionally depleted or overwhelmed. An experience of balance and peace is not something we attain, it is something we *reclaim*. And when we do, we feel at home in our bodies, more connected to our vitality, to our purpose, and to those around us.

You will discover that self-Reiki practice provides you with a compass for navigating through the complexities and uncertainties of life. This compass points us in the direction of well-being and resilience as we traverse the deep depths, narrow straits, as well as the passages through them. Self-Reiki mind-body skills are a natural, non-pharmacological, strengths-based approach to both (i) *building* resilience in order to sustain our ongoing well-being, and (ii) *utilizing* that resilience in moments of difficulty. Let's briefly explore the two faces of resilience, both of which Reiki self-practice addresses. When we think of resilience, what often comes to mind is the capacity to bounce back *after* adversity. While this is true, there is also another aspect. Resilience is not only *reacting* to challenges *after* they occur. Resilience involves purposefully *building* our own inner strengths, reserves, and capacities to feel courageous and whole despite disappointments, struggles, and social forces beyond our control. Resilience is not solely about claiming *our inner* qualities and wisdom, but also connecting with wisdom that lies in others.

We can all do our personal part in resilience building with self-Reiki practice. Yet, it is also true that we live in particular historical, social, cultural, political, and economic contexts that challenge our resilience-building capacity. One of the points this book makes is that what appears to be *individual-level* distress, such as anxiety, also occurs within the larger context of the social conditions that create it, such as inequality. We understand that the capacity for resilience resides not only *within* an individual. Rather, the capacity for resilience also depends on sociocultural, economic, and political resources available to people in their larger lifeworlds. These larger forces are out of the control of the individual. In such circumstances, we can't expect to meditate our way out of injustice, can we? So, then, what does Reiki practice offer in this case? Self-Reiki practice calms our nervous system, allowing us to be courageous; to think, speak, and act with wisdom and compassion so that we may pursue justice for ourselves and for all who are structurally disempowered. We can use this resilience as a resource for effectively confronting larger systemic brokenness, and creating the conditions for building a more peaceful and just world.

Self-Reiki practice is about facing uncertainty and relieving suffering of self and others. As you learn the Reiki practices outlined in this book you will find you can face uncertainty with greater courage and strength; loosen constriction; relate skillfully to your experiences; become more aware of your patterns and tendencies; and embody your authentic way of being in the world. Self-Reiki mind-body skills help us refocus our energy toward resilience, openness, and flexibility when faced with the unthinkable. What's more, as we cultivate our *own* state of well-being, we can create a peaceful space for *others* to experience. Self-Reiki practice helps us feel settled in ourselves, creating a ripple effect, enhancing our ability to be intentionally present for others, and even find ways to relieve the suffering of others. Self-Reiki practice allows us to live in peace with self and others.

Join us in learning some of the essential teachings and practices of Reiki for caring for yourself and living intentionally with heartfulness and mindfulness. Reiki self-practice is something no one else can do for us; we are the active agents in claiming our own growth and healing. While this book does not train or certify you as a Reiki practitioner, it does provide you with mind-body practices based in Reiki teachings that you can do for yourself. While many healing practices are solely practitioner-directed, Reiki practice is *both* practitioner-directed *and* self-directed. This book teaches you about the *self*-directed components of Reiki practice so you can optimally care for yourself. We encourage you to build self-Reiki practice time into your day to support you in claiming a greater sense of control and ease over how you relate to, and navigate through, what is happening inside and out. With self-Reiki practice we become aware first of the experience we are having; second, we become more aware of how we *relate to* the experience we are having; and third, we become more aware of how we are able to navigate through the experience with greater perspective, wisdom and compassion, enhancing our quality of life, and the quality of life around us.

Chapter 1, *The Questions*, answers the questions "What is Reiki?" and "How Does Reiki Heal?" Chapter 2, *The Roots*, presents the origins of the system of Reiki in Japan. In Chapter 3, *The Anchor*, you will learn the most essential Reiki meditative breathing practice, *hara* breathing, which anchors the body and cultivates a calm state of mind. Sitting in stillness with *hara* breathing is intertwined with what we term the Pause of nonreactivity, which is introduced in Chapter 4, *The Intentional Response*. We will then explore with you the fundamental Reiki meditations, *Joshin Kokyu-ho and Gassho* meditations, in Chapter 5, *The Spaciousness*. These meditations cultivate an enlarged perspective and spiritual expression.

The practice of hands-on self-healing is covered in Chapter 6, *The Hands*. Hands-on self-healing is a physical practice that allows us to listen to our inner self, and give ourselves the care that is necessary for healing. In Chapter 6, we also introduce the "Reiki Relief Remedy"; a hands-on-healing practice that can be used any time anxiety, worry, fear, or other forms of distress are experienced. Chapter 7, *The Centers of Awareness*, introduces you to the three Diamonds of *Ki*: the three centers of awareness in Japanese teachings – body, mind, and heart. Chapter 8, *The Compass*, draws you into the Reiki Precepts, a set of foundational principles of wise and purposeful living and being. In Chapter 9, *The Practice*, we provide some practical suggestions for establishing a sustainable self-Reiki practice for yourself. Chapter 10, *The Challenges*, describes ways in which self-Reiki practice can be supportive for specific populations and specific life challenges (in alphabetical order): adolescents, aging, burnout, children, illness, parenting, and relationships. Chapter 11, *The Social Suffering*, situates the place of self-Reiki practice in social justice work, enlarging the scope of healing beyond the individual. The final chapter, Chapter 12, *The Platform for Peace*, reminds us that self-Reiki practice is not only for when we are ill, but serves a salutogenic, or health-creating, purpose, supporting our well-being, aliveness, and spiritual growth. Throughout the chapters, we have interspersed anecdotes that illustrate the impact self-Reiki practice can have in our daily lives.

We invite you to embrace self-Reiki practice to create an inner terrain for yourself: a space of awareness; a space of resilience; a space of aliveness; a space in which there are many possibilities; a space overflowing with potential. You will find that the more you practice, the more you cultivate your inner resources to uplift and bring peace to self and others. We invite you to draw on Reiki practice for yourself so it becomes a natural part of your daily life in all its dimensions – physical, mental-emotional, and spiritual.

Chapter 1

The Questions: What is Reiki? How Does Reiki Heal?

What Is Reiki?

There are several ways to address the "What is Reiki" question and we will explore them here. Reiki practice is a holistic, complementary and integrative healing and meditation practice. Reiki practice supports and strengthens us holistically, and elicits a physiological healing response for mind, body, and emotions. The capacity to heal and feel whole lies within all of us. While Reiki self-practice is not designed to replace ongoing medical care, it can alleviate the many forms of distress that medical care may not fully address to help us reclaim aliveness and wholeness.

The system of Reiki refers to the practical and accessible mind-body-spirit healing and meditation teachings and practices developed by Mikao Usui in Japan in the 1920s, which then spread worldwide. These practices foster mindfulness and self-awareness of our thoughts and emotions. We all know that it is common to feel as if our minds are pulled in many directions, especially when we are under constant stress. We sometimes feel like our minds are on a runaway train! Our minds may be preoccupied by past regrets, losses, doubts, and disappointments; or leaping forward to the what-ifs. When we are gripped by fearful thoughts about past, present, and future, we can easily become overwhelmed and anxious. You will know your self-Reiki practice is indeed watering the seeds of healing when you tame the weeds of frantic overwhelm, and put the brakes on the runaway train of your mind. When we untangle the weeds, we create space to cultivate new growth, new possibilities, new spiritual connection, and even dimensions of ourselves that were hidden in the thicket.

The essence of Reiki practice is embodied in the Japanese concept, *shin shin kaizen*, meaning ongoing self-awareness and self-development; the internal process of discovering who we are and what is meaningful to us. With self-knowing, we can act in accord with our truest self. When we realize that our actions are in accord with our truest self, we are comfortable in our own skin and can feel whole. Because Reiki self-practice strengthens our capacity to be present with the reality of our experiences and our mind-state, we learn to trust ourselves to bring our everyday actions into alignment with our inner values. When the dissonance between our inner values and our outer actions is reduced, we are open to experience a new vibrancy. With this new vibrancy we may access spiritual expression that may have faded into to the background of our lives.

To fully understand what Reiki practice is, it is important to know the difference between healing and curing. Reiki is a *healing* system, in contrast to a curative system. To cure means to eliminate all evidence of disease; while to heal means to build and utilize one's inner qualities and skills to foster resilience, purpose, spiritual growth, and wholeness. Healing is salutogenic, as we create within ourselves the conditions for wellness. Even if one cannot be cured, one can still feel healed, or whole, with Reiki practice. Living with chronic illness that cannot be cured, for example, may bring with it feelings of hopelessness and fear. Reiki practice helps us claim the courage to stay present with the uncertainty and still live intentionally *with* purpose and *on* purpose, despite our difficulties.

Mikao Usui, who developed the system of Reiki in Japan, describes the essence of the Reiki teachings in this way:

The purpose of our lives is to achieve a peaceful and joyful mind-state, and then, while holding that peace within, realize our purpose. (cited in Hiroshi Doi 2014: 8-9, 103)

We learn from Usui's statement that Reiki teachings entail two processes: First, we cultivate our *inner* resources and qualities of well-being (*peaceful and joyful mind-state*). Second, we bring that peaceful and clear mind-state out into the world to fulfill our purpose and walk consciously in the world. To us, spirituality is all about living consciously and intentionally in accord with self, others, and the natural world; bringing a sacred outlook to what we say and do. Usui's statement reminds us that the healing benefits of self-Reiki practice extend far beyond the self. When *we're* feeling a peaceful and purposeful mind-body state, we are more aware of our capacity to be available to *others*, thereby enlarging our sphere of interaction, connection, and purpose. In our own ways, we can have a taste of the insight that Mikao Usui had on Mt. Kurama in Japan, when he said, *"I am in the Universe, and the Universe is within me."* We recognize that this mind-state is a stretch for us; no easy task. When we are confronted with acts of violence, racism, religious hatred, pervasive social and economic injustice, we may be at a loss as to how to make an impact. The hope is that, the more we practice Reiki mind-body skills, the more we can anchor ourselves in our courage to engage with the world in transformative ways: peace where there is violence; anti-racism where there is racism; inclusion where there is exclusion; and social and economic justice where there is injustice.

How Does Reiki Heal?

The main concept behind how Reiki heals is that, although the mind and body have built-in safeguards and repair mechanisms, when we are subject to continuous stressors, these mechanisms may become overtaxed, resulting in disease and illness. Reiki practice brings the body into a state of physiological rest and restorative relaxation, shifting the nervous system from sympathetic to parasympathetic. In other words, we can shift from feeling constricted or overwhelmed to calmer and more settled.

Quantitative and qualitative evidence [see Appendix for research papers] points to the fact that Reiki practice engages the body's natural healing capacity. The deep state of relaxation that Reiki facilitates acts through the autonomic nervous system to:

- regulate blood pressure and heart rate
- relieve tension and anxiety
- expand the ability of the immune system to defend against viruses and bacteria
- reduce inflammation
- stimulate the brain's production of endorphins that act to decrease the perception of pain and create a sense of well-being
- shift the brain waves from beta to alpha, indicative of deep, healing relaxation.

Let's understand the stress response. It is known that frequently activating the stress response inflicts long-term damage to our bodies. Stress researchers refer to allostatic load: the cumulative wear and tear of body and mind as a result of chronic stress (McEwen 1998; Picard, et al. 2016). Scientists have long known that stressful experiences *on their own* are not the sole cause of disease and illness; rather it's also our *responses* to stress that have the potential to create the terrain for, and susceptibility to, disease and distress (McEwen 1998). Our ability to cope with stress depends largely on how we experience it, relate to it, and what we can do to lessen its harmful effects. Constant anger, fear, and worry eat away at our immune system, whereas a calm, settled mind strengthens it. The mind is sometimes our own worst enemy because it has the capacity to ruin our days, our weeks, the months, and even years of our lives, with its rumination and constant worry. Rumination and worry send chemical messages throughout our bodies that can compromise our physical and emotional health and well-being.

Reiki practice can help lessen the harmful effects of stress that bring suffering to body and mind. We define suffering as "severe distress associated with events that threaten the intactness of the person" (Cassell 1982). You may recall the earlier discussion about how Reiki practice brings about healing, wholeness and intactness. As such, Reiki mind-body practices directly address our experience of suffering. Self-Reiki practice provides skills for regulating our attention and energy. These skills are an antidote to the harmful consequences of stress that cause us pain and suffering. As we down-regulate the nervous system, we settle our minds, bodies, and emotions. In this calmer state, we are able to tend to our thoughts and feelings with awareness. With this self-awareness, we can notice any harmful habitual patterns that bring us suffering and do not support our well-being. Reiki practice not only helps us *become aware* that we are in the grip of a habitual stress response, Reiki mind-body practices also assist us in *softening* our suffering and reaching for wholeness and intactness. When we are mindful of how we relate to stressful circumstances, we create an opening to ease, and can lessen the physiological stress response. Further, we can strengthen our Reiki mind-body skills throughout our lives, making self-Reiki a lifelong practice that promotes self-regulation, resilience, wholeness, and spiritual growth in the face of stress and adversity. The Reiki meditative *hara* breathing practice we introduce in Chapter 4, for example, is a way we can ease our suffering, and touch our aliveness, instead of fueling our suffering.

Let's face it, life gets messy, uncomfortable, painful, confusing; and we struggle and suffer. We often find ourselves gripped by intense thoughts and feelings. In the clutch of anxious thoughts we can also become stuck in a constricted, repetitive story. The practice of Reiki has been shown to help people feel less gripped by their anxious thoughts. By calming mind and body,

Reiki practice helps us express our spiritual selves as we enlarge our field of vision beyond our constricted, repetitive story, and envision possibilities and actions we could not perceive before.

Beyond this, when we experience marginalized identities and encounter ongoing racial, religious, gender, sex, disability, or other bias and harm, we can experience profound anxiety, adversity, and trauma. While Reiki practice itself may not appear to directly address the drivers of such harm, Reiki practice *can* support caring for ourselves and others even in the midst of such adversity. Reiki self-practice supports us to find a platform of courage to take action in the midst of troubling sociopolitical forces and circumstances.

Self-Reiki practice helps with anxiety-provoking situations which arise in our lives, whether these are ongoing chronic stressful situations or unexpected shocks that life presents. The healing process is not a straight line; we may take two steps forward and one step back, and even one step sideways, but we can always go inward reclaiming our courage and steadiness even when we feel unsure and scared. The more we practice self-Reiki, though, the more we become self-aware of our mind-body state. The feelings of helplessness from the disappointments, harms, and uncertainties of life may be eased as we rediscover an inner foundation of courage and self-awareness on which to relate our experiences. Our Reiki healing process can therefore bring us to a more resilient and peaceful mind-body state even as we face hardships in our lives.

Join us in a reflection: What does living with courage and resilience look and feel like for you.

- *Sitting comfortably in this moment, gently acknowledging a current situation of uncertainty or hurt, and gently just dipping a toe into the feelings.*
- *Exploring with caring curiosity any feelings (anxiety, sadness, fear, or anger, for example) that may rise and fall; allowing these*

to come and go. Knowing it is safe to sit with these feelings for a moment without judging them or needing to change them.

- *Beginning now to create a movie in your mind of what it looks like to trust yourself to stand on a solid platform as feelings are simply allowed to be felt with warmth for yourself.*
- *Pausing and noticing what it can feel like to fuel resilience, and inner strength. For by sitting with uncomfortable thoughts and emotions that is exactly what you are doing – cultivating courage.*

When we take the time to envision ourselves in this way, we become aware of new possibilities for relating to our experiences with courage and purposefulness.

We can sum up the intent of how Reiki practice heals in two words, one of which is a Japanese word. The two words are: *Misogi* and expansion. *Misogi* means purification or cleansing; our minds feel clearer, refreshed, more intact, and less cluttered. The second word, expansion, is about creating inner spaciousness in which we enlarge our capacity to mindfully accommodate the experiences and people in our lives. When we feel clear, whole, and centered on the inside (*misogi*), we create an expansive space to participate more fully in the flow of life (expansion).

We can all build this mind-body-spirit healing state with the practices introduced in this book. Even for a moment right now, once again, we invite you to engage in a mind-body-spirit experience of the concepts of *misogi* and expansion.

- *Feel yourself landing here now in a way that feels solid and settled to you.*
- *Allowing a sense of softening.*
- *Breathing in and sensing, or intending, ease within yourself. That is misogi.*
- *Breathing out a slow, lengthened breath and sensing, or intending, an expansive spaciousness infused with awareness of*

beauty and the sacred in the everyday. That is expansion; that is spiritual expression.

The key to wellbeing is to be able to understand that things are uncertain. It is not our job to make things certain.

No one can. The secret is to understand that things are uncertain and then live with dignity and beauty in the midst of it.

When we do so we move into less struggle, less fear, and greater ease, wisdom, and resilience.

– Jack Kornfield

Wholeness is the goal, but wholeness does not mean perfection.
– Parker Palmer

Chapter 2

The Roots: The Origins of Reiki

We welcome you into the rich historical and cultural context that lies behind the development of the system of Reiki in Japan. Mikao Usui, who developed *Usui Reiki Ryoho* (*Usui System of Natural Healing*), was born on August 15, 1865 in southern Japan during the Meiji Restoration. It was during this time that Japan opened its borders after 200 years of isolation, ushering in modernization, urbanization, and industrialization (Stiene 2005: 5). These rapid economic changes also brought social change to Japan, and people seemed to have felt a need for deeper meaning and purpose. This search for meaning, purpose, and spiritual expression was already embodied by Usui in his Buddhist studies and practice (Stiene 2005: 5).

In his ongoing spiritual searching, Usui spent three years on a meditation retreat at a Kyoto Zen Temple in 1919, followed by an experience of *anshin ritsumei*, or awakening, in 1922 while on Mt. Kurama (Petter 2012: 44). An experience of *anshin ritsumei* entails committing one's life to wisdom and compassion, staying settled and solid, without attachment to success or failure. After his Mt. Kurama experience, Usui came to a deep realization that, *"I am in the Universe and the Universe is within me."* This reflects a participation consciousness – a spiritual mind-state in which we partake of, and contribute to, all life. All of us can experience this participation consciousness, as Usui did, as it is part of the human potential. Even when suffering, adversity, and harm are part of our history and current circumstances, we can touch that human potential within us all.

Following his experience on Mt. Kurama, Mikao Usui set up a *dojo* (a place of learning and teaching) in Tokyo called *Usui Reiki Ryoho Gakkai* (Usui Natural Healing Society). Usui's teachings included meditation and healing practices. On September 1, 1923, a devastating earthquake, the Great Kano Earthquake with a magnitude of 7.9, struck the Tokyo-Yokohama metropolitan area on the main island of Honshu. The death toll was estimated to have exceeded 140,000; with 180,000 people injured, and 1.5 million people left homeless (Petter 2012: 54). According to information on Usui's Memorial Stone, "feeling pity for the survivors, [Usui] went out every morning... and saved an innumerable number of people" ("Lessons from the Usui Mikao Memorial Stone," Stiene 2008). The reputation of *Usui Reiki Ryoho* spread in part as a result of Usui's work with earthquake survivors.

Usui began traveling throughout Japan teaching and practicing Reiki. During this time, Usui experienced two strokes, and it has been reported that he was able to heal himself of their after-effects, and continue practicing and teaching (Petter 2012: 59). Later, while traveling in Hiroshima, Usui died of a cerebral hemorrhage after a stroke on March 9, 1926 (Petter 2012: 58). Usui was buried at the Saihoji Temple in Tokyo (ibid).

The system of Reiki was introduced to the US from Japan in 1938 by Hawayo Takata, and, thereafter, spread throughout the world. In most countries, including the US, the traditional Japanese practices have been modified and may not reflect the traditional practices that originated in Japan. In this book we introduce you to the Japanese Reiki practices that we have researched and learned from our teachers and mentors. Reiki is currently offered in hospitals, hospices, wellness centers, support groups, community settings, and in private practitioner settings across the US and the world as a complement to medical care and treatment.

When we engage in our self-Reiki practices, we can experience a taste of Usui's *anshin ritsumei* by reducing the weight of judgment of self and others; of our likes and dislikes. In this way we can cultivate a mind that is open and expansive, anchored by a body that is steady and solid. We are available to both ourselves and others.

Join us in Chapters 3-8 as we introduce the self-Reiki mind-body skills and practices that strengthen and support us so we can be at peace with ourselves and others. The essential self-Reiki practices you will learn are:

- *Hara* breathing (Ch. 3), which is a simple and natural breathing practice that elicits a shift from the sympathetic to parasympathetic nervous system.
- The Pause (Ch. 4), which helps us put the brakes on our emotional reactivity.
- *Joshin Kokyu-ho* and *Gassho* meditations (Ch. 5) that anchor and focus our scattered minds and invite in a spacious openness and spiritual connection.
- Hands-on self-Reiki practice (Ch. 6), including the "Reiki Relief Remedy," which allows us to care for ourselves in a compassionate way, and brings about a physiological relaxation response.
- The Three Diamonds of *Ki* – three centers of awareness of body, mind, and heart – are introduced (Ch. 7), along with associated meditations.
- The Reiki Precepts (Ch. 8), which are a set of teachings, or principles, that brings us into alignment with our deepest values.

Chapter 3

The Anchor: *Hara* Breathing Practice

Visualize for a moment a palm tree in the midst of a tropical storm. We have all seen news images of this: the upper branches and leaves of the palm tree wildly tossed about by the rains and winds. However, if the news camera were to lower its lens to the base of the palm tree, we would see stillness where the tree trunk is rooted to the ground. Nothing is turbulent or unsettled at the base of the tree, yet at the same time, the trunk solidly holds what is happening above it. This visual points to an experience available to all of us. We invite you to hold this visual in your mind as you learn the first meditative practice, *hara* breathing.

One of the most essential Reiki meditative practices is *hara* breathing. *Hara* breathing is a straightforward and uncomplicated breathing practice that allows us to claim peace with self and others. *Hara* (also known as *tanden* or *lower dantian*) is a Japanese word referring to a center of awareness conceptually located in the lower abdomen, three finger-widths below the navel, in the exact center of the body. The *hara* is a space of awareness that knows no bounds, as it connects us with both self and all things and all beings (Wilberg 2011). The *hara* involves our entire being as it anchors and centers body, mind, and emotions in steadiness. *Hara* is the stable platform on which we stand, and from which flow intentionality, mindfulness, spaciousness, and a participation consciousness with all that is. It is central to everything in life that when we feel an inner stability, we can enlarge our capacity to stay in connection with our own experiences and with all beings around us.

Practicing *hara* breathing is a natural way for us to have an impact on our own body's physiology, eliciting a shift from the sympathetic to the parasympathetic nervous system. *Hara* breathing enables us to recalibrate the systems of our body toward a state of calm and dynamic well-being. This breathing practice is a skill for emotional well-being, allowing us to get in touch with our thoughts and feelings, including those that are uncomfortable. At the same time, as we continue to connect with ourselves through *hara* breathing, we can experience our strength, aliveness and vitality. Physiologically, *hara* breathing activates the vagus nerve, which signals the brain, heart, lungs, and digestive tract to rest and restore. *Hara* breathing is a key to managing our state of mind and stress level because when we practice *hara* breathing we signal the vagus nerve to activate the calming parasympathetic branch of our nervous system. With this simple and effective practice of *hara* breathing, we bring balance and wholeness to body and mind. This is neither a state of dullness nor of blissing out; rather it is a state of connection to our vibrancy and essence, alongside a settled mind-body.

Imagine a phone call coming in unexpectedly at 10:30am and it is from a loved one's school or workplace. Our immediate emotional and physiological reaction of worry or fear elicits the sympathetic nervous system, and we are in fight or flight mode. Although this is natural, we also have the capacity to steady our brain's perceptions and reactions to not only this particular situation, but to whatever may come at us throughout the day, pleasant or unpleasant.

Isn't it wonderful and amazing that we can support, soothe, and nourish our own nervous system? Let's preview the how-tos of *hara* breathing: In *hara* breathing practice, we breathe in a refreshing breath through the nose, with the intent that the breath travels all the way down the body to the *hara* space. When we are ready to exhale (through the nose or the mouth), we allow the out-breath to comfortably and gently last a little longer than the in-breath. The lengthened expansive out-breath signals the brain to calm and settle mind and body; down-regulating our nervous system from sympathetic to parasympathetic mode.

With *hara* breathing we get in touch with our body, mind, and spirit. By breathing slowly into the lower abdomen (*hara*), and gradually lengthening and expanding the out-breath, we skillfully rest our awareness on the qualities within ourselves of being strong, rooted, and resilient, like the trunk of the palm tree.

This practice of pausing and connecting to our inner stillness through *hara* breathing does *not* mean we push away troubling thoughts and feelings. Rather, when we practice *hara* breathing, we discover we can create an inner space to *sit with* uncomfortable thoughts and emotions, and be less gripped by them as they arise. Similarly, in yoga practice *"asana"* means to "sit with what comes up."

Think, for a moment, about a crying baby. By crying, the baby is communicating something, some need, some discomfort. We have to be with the crying baby, soothing and comforting the child with warmth and understanding. Similarly, we have to be with our thoughts, feelings, and physical sensations in the same way. Our own thoughts, feelings, and physical sensations are communicating with us. When we practice *hara* breathing, we are practicing staying with what comes up, paying attention to it, even if it is distressing. Instead of running away and trying to escape from unpleasant thoughts and feelings, *hara* breathing creates an inner spaciousness. In this space, we connect to awareness and courage, trusting ourselves to be with strong emotions, and that these will come and go. Our *hara* breathing practice inspires an awareness that we don't have to run from ourselves with restlessness and constant busy-ness.

Our society promotes busy-ness and running for the next big thing. This makes it easy to fall into the trap of avoiding or burying any unpleasant thoughts and feelings. As we develop our *hara* breathing practice we are able to tend to our uncomfortable thoughts and feelings, instead of running away from them, which ultimately weakens our reserves. *Hara* breathing encourages a healing and caring relationship with our troubling thoughts and feelings. When we hang in there with our difficult thoughts and feelings, instead of running from them, lo and behold, we discover that we can make room for them. This has been referred to as "putting out the welcome mat" to the thoughts and feelings that come up, so we can relate with care to our experiences as they truly are.

Breathing into the *hara* calms the mind, regulates the emotions, and relaxes the body so we can build a secure and strong foundation; rooted, like a palm tree in a storm. With that solid foundation, our minds are clearer, calmer, and more focused instead of frantic, racing, and scattered. With this sense of calm we can navigate through the fears, worries and uncertainties in our lives with greater resilience, yet with a softness and tenderness that comes from feeling settled within. From this place of greater emotional stability, we can create a calm, comforting presence for ourselves and for those around us. The in-breath nourishes and refreshes us with vitality and aliveness. The expansive out-breath reminds us to be open-minded and flexible when difficulties come up. With *hara* breathing's lengthened, expansive out-breath, our experience of life enlarges as we open up the self to the world; we discover we have space and tenderness within us. We experience in *hara* breathing that the inner determines the outer. In fact, this is precisely the state of mind we seek to embody with our self-Reiki practice. There is no medication that can anchor us in the *hara*, strengthen our inner resources for resilience, allow our minds to clear, and encourage and inspire our hearts to open. This is why growing our self-Reiki meditation and healing practice – a natural approach to healing mind and body – is so essential to our well-being.

We can *be* the base of the palm tree, even in the midst of life's storms. No matter what stormy uncertainties our lives may bring at any given point, the practice of *hara* breathing can anchor us. How is *hara* breathing helpful? Because in the middle of life's storms, troubling thoughts grip us, causing us to unravel as the sympathetic nervous system takes over. Therefore, it is very important to remind ourselves to anchor ourselves with *hara* breathing, allowing a shift to the parasympathetic nervous system. When we practice *hara* breathing we create a space of potential and possibilities; an opportunity to access our inner strength and wisdom. We nourish ourselves at that very moment in time.

Anecdote: *Very few things in life can compare to the sheer terror of sitting in a waiting room for the results of one's one-year post-diagnosis cancer screening. In the specific case of mammograms, which may require additional views, Josephina, a breast cancer survivor, may be waiting for 2-3 hours, watching other patients get cleared to leave. The dread sets in that there must be something seriously wrong. What can Josephina do to ease her body and mind? Even in the midst of the anguish of waiting and the fear of the unknown, Josephina can practice hara breathing to get through each agonizing moment of trepidation. Josephina, of course, is aware that hara breathing practice will not change the outcome of the medical test, yet it certainly helps immensely to get through the waiting.* How amazing it is that we can rely on ourselves and our *hara* breathing as a mind-body skill to get us through the really tough moments in our lives. When we are in a totally vulnerable situation, being able to rely on our own breath bestows upon us the gift of caring for ourselves.

The Practice of *Hara* Breathing:

We gently suggest that, in order to maintain your sustainable Reiki self-practice, you set a timer for 5-15 minutes, or longer.

- *Landing here now, settling your body in a comfortable position.*
- *Noticing any tension you may be holding in your body – head, jaw, neck, shoulders, hips, legs, feet – and seeing if it can be*

eased. If it cannot, then saying to yourself, "I am sitting with some tension in my _____ right now, and that's okay."
- *Closing your eyes, or gazing toward the floor approximately 3 feet away from you.*
- *Bringing your focus to your breath. Noticing the breath coming in and going out.*
- *Begin to slow down your breath. Sensing and embracing the stillness.*
- *While being mindful of the breath, experiencing, or sensing, a refreshing breath coming in through the nose, with the intent that the breath is carried all the way down to the hara.*
- *When the breath is ready to be released, allowing the out-breath (through the nose or mouth) to last a little longer than the in-breath.*
- *For those who prefer to count the breath, consider starting with a count of 4 on the in-breath and 6-8 on the out-breath.*
- *Becoming aware of your body settling and calming.*
- *Your in-breath and out-breath are working in harmony and wholeness without force or hard work, or concern about doing it "right."*
- *Allowing a refreshing breath in.*
- *Allowing a lengthened breath out.*

Continue with *hara* breathing and it will support and encourage inner steadiness, balance, and wholeness from which we can soften and ultimately express a sacred outlook in our lives.

While this essential Reiki meditative practice may seem to be solitary, over time *hara* breathing practice expands from a private meditative experience to a capacity to truly give space and listen to others. When we practice *hara* breathing and become accustomed to sitting with our *own* thoughts and feelings, we also connect to our capacity to sit with *other* people and *their* thoughts and feelings. In this way, we embody deep, compassionate listening to others. This is healing to others as it encourages others to freely share their experiences, and feel validated and whole despite their hardships. You can see that *hara* breathing is designed to be healing for both self and others.

> *No one can be successful in the art of meditation without having passed the gate of breathing.*
> – Thich Nhat Hanh

Chapter 4

The Intentional Response: The Mindful Pause

When we invite a mindful pause into any moment, we can bring awareness to our heart-mind (*kokoro*) in that moment. The word *kokoro* is a Japanese word for both mind and heart at the same time. So when we practice a Mindful Pause it is one and the same as a Heartful Pause. Similarly, mindfulness in Japanese is *nen*, meaning the heart and mind come together into this very moment. The value of a mindful/heartful pause is to restore emotional regulation and create an inner spaciousness. The Pause is a deliberate, physical pause we can take in any moment to allow the mind to gather us in so we can attend to, and tend to, our heart/mind-state in the moment. The Pause helps us become less reactive to stressors as we create some space between the event and our response. By creating a gap, we can bring our experience back under our own control and realize we have a choice in how we respond; that is emotional freedom. Each time we give ourselves that Pause, that gap, we shift our view of ourselves; of how we relate to our thoughts, feelings and experiences.

In Zen teachings, a teacher was asked, "What is the teaching of an entire lifetime?" His answer: "An appropriate response" (Lesser 2019: 67). So how we respond intentionally and consciously to life circumstances and people is a primary task of our lives. This chapter guides you to experience this mindful Pause for yourself during everyday interactions and situations so you can reach for an "appropriate response" and feel a deeper, more authentic, connection to your experiences and interactions.

Why do we need this Pause? This Pause is necessary in order to create a space of calm for ourselves in which to reclaim both ease and our inner wisdom. We all have habitual ways of reacting based on the conditionings from our culture, our upbringing, and our unique past experiences. Over the course of our lives, these reactive habits become our default mode; like being on auto-pilot. When we are in automatic mode we are effectively being highjacked by the part of the brain that controls our emotions and impulses (the limbic system). When we *don't* take time to Pause and tend to mind and body, we are apt to go directly into this default mode and react with old patterns of behavior that we may regret. In this default mode, we may become agitated or constricted. Further, a constricted, tense, or agitated mind-body state is associated with the sympathetic fight-flight response. We need this Pause of mindful awareness to loosen the constriction and to anchor our entire being in the moment so we can call on our strengths and respond with awareness, compassion and patience in both uniquely difficult situations and in everyday moments. This definitely takes practice and persistence, as we learn to acknowledge the inner tensions that come up for us every day.

As we become more mindful of our bodies, thoughts, and emotions, we can ask ourselves: What are my thoughts? Is my mind working for me or against me? How can I find a strong anchor within? A helpful practice here is to gently inquire into ourselves: "What do I really want to pay attention to at this moment?" When we pay attention, we may come to recognize, for example, that fear lies at the core of our reactive agitation or constriction (Leitch, Social-Resilience Model). We recognize that when we are in a fear-response, our knee-jerk reaction may be to lash out or become defensive. When we Pause, though, and consciously become aware that fear is driving us, we can intentionally reach for "an appropriate response."

How do we take this Pause, especially in moments of upset? We Pause by making a conscious *choice* to tend to our inner state in the moment, so we can put the brakes on our auto-pilot reactions. It is necessary to condition ourselves over and over again so that Pausing becomes part of who we are. It is like muscle conditioning, and this time we are strengthening the muscle of mindfulness. It's a discipline; the more we practice, the more natural Pausing becomes, and the more we strengthen our self-awareness and our "appropriate response." The more we practice the Pause, the more familiar we become with *how* to do it and how to make it work for us. Each time we Pause we are rewiring our brains toward greater stability, well-being, spaciousness, and emotional freedom. We soon learn that this practice is about creating a Pause-space of stillness in the moment so we can become mindful of our reactions. The cumulative benefit of practicing Pausing when upset is that it is a natural way to root ourselves in our inner strengths while staying mindful of our habitual hasty reactions so we can respond more thoughtfully.

When we put on the brakes, we give ourselves a breather in which to pay attention to thoughts and feelings bubbling up in the moment. Pausing grants us the self-control to interrupt our hasty words and actions in the moment. We find we can actually pivot from our knee-jerk reaction to more mindful and heartful action. Wisdom from spiritual teachers, including Jack Kornfield, among others, instructs this helpful practice for ushering in a mindful and heartful Pause: We can silently ask ourselves, "What would love have me say and do today?" and invite a Pause to reflect on our "appropriate response."

Here are some tips for how to put the brakes on our emotional reactivity and access the Pause:

- *Bringing your full awareness to the types of situations that may cause your knee-jerk reactions.*
- *Now imagining yourself in one of those situations, but this time you prepare yourself to Pause.*
- *Possibly ask yourself: "What would love have me say and do at*

this time?"

- *Visualizing being like the base of a palm tree in a storm.*
- *Sensing that your mind and body can settle down, like the snow in a snow globe.*
- *Inviting your body to feel solid and stable like a mountain that accommodates all of the seasonal changes that take place on it.*
- *Coaching yourself to bring clarity and patience to the moment.*
- *Softening the heart, feeling yourself open to possibilities.*
- *Moving forward patiently, responding with mindfulness and heartfulness.*

By practicing these Pause tips, we can bypass our default mode and become steady and composed, open and available; strengthening our ability to respond mindfully with wisdom and compassion.

In what life situations might the mindful Pause be most helpful? We bring you five brief real-life scenarios in which practicing the Pause of nonreactivity has been helpful to us and those we know for living in peace with ourselves and others.

We nickname the first situation, *"Jump In & Fix."* This is when we are emotionally invested in another person's well-being, and want to jump in and fix every problem for them. But when we are driven by our own fearful feelings to jump in to fix their problem, it may sometimes do more harm than good. Pausing can settle our intense emotions, creating a space for problem-solving and supportive collaboration to unfold without the need to leap in to "fix" another person. In fact, Pausing to access *our* composure allows the other person to find and speak *their* truth, thereby honoring our being *and* their being. When we Pause in nonreactivity we allow space and freedom for others to be themselves.

Anecdote: *Lee was recently laid off from their job. Their sister, Cecelia, was very concerned for Lee's well-being and rushed in for the* *rescue. Cecelia came over to Lee's place unannounced, armed with job search information, ready to fix Lee's situation. "I've got this covered, Lee," Cecelia proclaimed. "That job wasn't good for you anyway, and here's what you need to do now..." Cecelia continued on and on, even as Lee took a step back and turned away. Seeing Lee's reaction, Cecelia then realized she had to Pause and give Lee the space and freedom to express their thoughts and feelings. Lee was not interested in hearing about job search tips, rather they wanted to talk about the experience of their job loss. Cecelia then realized that Pausing had a more affirming impact than pushing.* Cecelia was able to Pause in stillness, experience composure, restrain her anxiety, and give Lee the space to express their truth.

A second set of circumstances in which to practice the Pause is what we term the *"Personal Affront."* This may occur when our sense of worth as a capable person feels threatened. Think about what you consider the core of what you do and who you are. Now imagine someone calls all of that into question. Our knee-jerk reaction may be to take the criticism as a hurtful attack and lash out. If, however, we were to Pause and settle our nervous system, we could assess the remarks with discernment instead of automatically experiencing them as an affront to our self-worth. Pausing in this way, we equip ourselves to assess the situation clearly and really listen to the other person.

Anecdote: *A college teacher is approached by a student after class. "Hey, professor, that last exam was completely unfair and I do not deserve this grade." The professor feels like she was hit in the gut, because she had given the exam questions ahead of time. Nonetheless, her knee-jerk reaction was to feel diminished, question her skills and competency. But when the professor shifted her reactivity into the Pause, she was able to create the necessary space to become aware of her inner state. In this way she was able to focus on the student's needs, instead of on her own hurt feelings. She listened patiently to the student's concerns, considered the student's perspective, and worked*

in partnership for a solution that met both her and her student's needs.
Both felt emotionally freer to move forward.

"*Feeling Helpless*" is the third opportunity where mindful Pausing is invaluable. These are situations in which we feel there is nothing we can do to make things better. We may feel helpless, anxious, and even angry, with no control over a situation. When we think there is nothing we can do, though, that is not really true! Even in extremely distressing situations, the Pause *is* the gift we can give to ourselves and others. When we Pause we can stay present with ourselves and with our own feelings. Further, when we Pause and claim composure, we realize that we can be available to others and *their* experiences. Being present to another *is* our essential offering.

Anecdote: *Alan makes a weekly visit to his cousin, Thomas, in a nursing facility. Thomas has been living with ALS for over a year. Early on, Alan did everything he could to make things more comfortable for his cousin. As time went on, however, Alan struggled with the fact that he was helpless to do anything to make things better for Thomas. Over the months, Alan noticed that if he Paused and gained composure, he did not have to fuel those feelings of helplessness. When he Paused, Alan's focus shifted away from his own anxiety and feelings of helplessness. Alan became more steady, his mind was able to calm, and his emotions to settle. The more Alan practiced the Pause of nonreactivity outside of his visits to Thomas, as well as during the visits, the more mindful of his feelings he became. As he became more aware and intentionally present, Alan could appreciate the time with Thomas, and their visits become more peaceful.* When Alan steadied himself, he realized he had become fixated on his *own* anxious feelings. This prevented him from being open to what might be possible during these visits. He experienced that his intentional presence *was* enough.

The fourth scenario, "*Opposing Viewpoints,*" occurs when we find ourselves in situations where people have differing viewpoints, each trying to convince the other that *their* perspective is correct. Each individual, as well as the group dynamic as a whole, becomes emotionally charged, as each person tries to prove their point. The argument takes on a momentum of its own, escalating as people get vehemently stuck to their stance, stubbornly refusing to listen to others. Imagine the difference it would make if just one or two people put on the brakes and Paused? What would be brought into the space? When one person pauses with nonreactivity, they bring their receptivity and their availability into the space. By Pausing and gaining composure, they de-escalate the situation, and create the optimal conditions for listening and then they can really hear other people's positions, and move forward to a resolution.

Anecdote: *The town of Portsham was at an impasse over how to best use a recently bequeathed parcel of land in the town. The voice of one bloc was adamant that the land should become a park, as public park space was severely limited in Portsham. The opposing bloc vehemently disagreed, arguing that a public park would only cost the town money. Instead this bloc pushed for a municipal metered parking lot since it would bring in revenue and the location was convenient to the town center. The most recent town meeting was filled with contentious debate, screaming, raised fists, and finger-pointing. Joe had to step out of the fray because he felt he was going to burst out with something he would regret. He then remembered his Reiki mind-body skills, Paused, and took several deep hara breaths. Joe could feel his entire system down-regulating: his hot head and flushed face cooling down; his pounding heart rate slowing. He could feel himself becoming steady, settled, and anchored in his body. In this state of composure, Joe returned to the meeting and reached out to the mayor, suggesting an idea of how to build consensus.* When we approach controversy with a steady body and mind, we can see possibilities that were hidden to us when we were agitated. The Pause fosters renewed awareness which not only helps ourselves, but also helps everyone around us collaborate to solve conflict. When we nurture an inner calm by practicing the Pause, we can cultivate not only self-growth, but also collective growth.

The last situation, *"Unexpected Behavior,"* is when we are caught off guard by the unexpected behavior of others. This may range from harmful outbursts that appear to come out-of-the-blue, to suddenly-disclosed information that was previously concealed. In some of these situations, we may feel mind-body overwhelm: head spinning, stomach churning, breath constricting. In other situations, we may feel crushing devastation: legs like Jello, heartbroken, head stunned. No matter the situation, when we practice the Pause, we can take the necessary space to anchor ourselves in our body so we can move through the period of overwhelm and distress intact.

Anecdote: *Reid was sitting in his car parked in the lot of a busy grocery store when another driver backed into his car. He got out of his car and approached the driver, who was still sitting in his car. "Excuse me, you just hit my car." Reid was shocked by the unexpected vehement retort of, "No I didn't; that dent was there before." Reid said, "No, I was sitting in my car and directly saw you back into the side of my car door." The driver opened his car door with rage and stood up threateningly, fists waving at Reid's face. Reid jumped back in his car and locked the door. The other driver drove away. Reid wished he had had the wherewithal to have taken a picture of the driver's license plate and called the police. However, Reid was frozen and unable to take action.* If Reid had been able to access an inner steadiness by Pausing, he may have been able to have his wits about him and address the unexpected and intimidating outburst with "an appropriate response."

Summary of the benefits of practicing the Pause for self and others:

Benefits for the Self. A mindful Pause is critical to our own health and well-being. We nurture our own well-being when we Pause. When we don't Pause, we can get stuck in a harmful stress response which has serious negative impacts on our well-being. As noted in Chapter 1, our emotional reactivity is linked with the stress response, and may foster chronic inflammation; increased blood pressure and heart rate; decreased immune function; and increased sensitivity to pain. Beyond the physical level, Pausing is *emotionally* self-rewarding. When we mindfully Pause we feel better about ourselves because we realize we can control our responses to other people and situations. Ultimately, the ongoing benefit to the self is that the more we practice the Pause, the more ease-filled, balanced, and steady our mind-body state becomes, and the more emotionally free we feel. On the level of spirit, a mindful Pause expands our vision of what is possible and brings us into compassionate presence with self and others.

Benefits for Others. Practicing the Pause benefits not only our *own* well-being, but the well-being of those around us. When we nurture our *own* well-being by practicing the Pause, we soften ourselves, and draw on our patience and kindness to be available to others. This allows *them* the silence, space, and freedom to be themselves. Remember the Zen teaching about the lesson of a lifetime being developing and refining appropriate response? We benefit *others* with our appropriate response because we can restore equilibrium to a fraught interaction or situation, mend ruptures in our relationships, and feel deep authentic connection with others.

Chapter 5

The Spaciousness: *Joshin Kokyu-ho* and *Gassho* Meditations

Joshin Kokyu-Ho

The teachings of Reiki include the meditation known in Japanese as *Joshin Kokyu-ho*. *Joshin Kokyu-ho* can be translated as "the cleansing breath to stabilize mind and body." *Joshin Kokyu-ho* builds on *hara* breathing practice, and deepens our capacity for creating spaciousness. Practicing *Joshin Kokyu-ho* meditation has two intentions: First, the practice anchors the scattered, agitated, busy mind by steadying body, mind, and emotions through the breath. Second, the practice of *Joshin Kokyu-ho* enlarges our *kokoro* (heart-mind) to create spaciousness. Spaciousness is the spiritual experience of transcending the feeling of constriction in our *kokoro*. *Joshin Kokyu-ho* helps us steady mind and body because spaciousness and open-mindedness can only come from a stable core.

Let's imagine a snow globe. We shake it up and love seeing the "snow" floating around the little scene within the globe. But can we see the scene clearly when the snow is scattered about? Of course not, it is obscured and unclear. We are like the snow globe. When our mind is tangled in knots we cannot see clearly, but when the "snow" of the mind settles, we can see things as they truly are.

When we practice *Joshin Kokyu-ho* we claim an inner space in the *hara* in which to settle our thoughts and emotions, like the "snow" in the snow globe. In that stillness, we become grounded and clear. When we practice *Joshin Kokyu-ho*, there are physiological benefits as well: we are signaling the brain to down-regulate physical and emotional hyper-arousal, just like the "snow" settles in the snow globe. When we practice

Joshin Kokyu-ho, we anchor and stabilize the runaway train of our minds. When the mind is clear and calm, we are better able to navigate through the commotion of life with a more solid, steady self. The solid, steady self sees things as they truly are, instead of jumping to erroneous conclusions, even when life gets complicated and messy.

Each time we inhale a cleansing *ki*-filled breath, we bring mindful awareness to the path of the breath as it moves down into the *hara* space. With this in-breath we anchor the mind in the body, feeling grounded and centered in the present moment. With the out-breath, we sense our settled, refreshed self expanding and opening outward into our surroundings. From this place of solidity we can feel spaciousness, an open-mindedness, an open-heartedness, and spiritual expression. As our anchored self expands outward, we create a space of peace for not only ourselves, but for others as well.

The more we practice the in-breath of *Joshin Kokyu-ho*, the more we can bring our mind back into our body and under control, so that we don't get tossed about by our thoughts. When the mind is united with the body through the in-breath, we are anchored in the present moment. The in-breath of *Joshin Kokyu-ho* requires us to always come back to the breath and the body. Each in-breath through the body exists only in the present moment, unlike our thoughts which may be stuck in the past or race to the future. The very physicality of the in-breath almost "tricks" us into feeling naturally awake to the present moment. The more we practice the out-breath of *Joshin Kokyu-ho*, the more the mind-body-breath connection we have created allows us to soften the *kokoro* and open the self to the world. This expansive out-breath enlarges our capacity to create a soulful spaciousness of reciprocity and responsibility between ourselves and all beings. Our practice of *Joshin Kokyu-ho* settles us like the snow in the snow globe while, at the same time, broadening our consciousness.

The Practice of *Joshin Kokyu-Ho*:

- *Landing here now, settling your body in a comfortable position. Noticing any tension you may be holding in your body – head, jaw, neck, shoulders, hips, legs, or feet – and seeing if it can be eased. If it cannot, then saying to yourself, "I am sitting with some tension in my _____ right now."*
- *Resting your hands comfortably on your lap with palms downward or upward.*
- *Closing your eyes or gazing at the floor approximately 3 feet away from you.*
- *Bringing awareness to your breath. Noticing the breath coming in and going out. Beginning to gently lengthen your out-breath without force.*
- *As you inhale, experience a refreshing ki-filled breath through the nose all the way down to the hara. Allowing your awareness to follow the path of the breath, settling the mind down into the hara space and the body, like the snow in the snow globe.*
- *On the lengthened out-breath, experiencing your refreshed self expanding and opening out from your entire being in all directions into your surroundings.*
- *Experiencing yourself as open-minded and open-hearted, and as spacious as your out-breath; overcoming constriction, feeling your mind-state liberated.*

Joshin Kokyu-ho, the cleansing breath to stabilize mind and body, allows us to relate to the present moment with freshness, grounded openness and awareness, and to share that state of being with others around us.

Gassho Meditation

Gassho Meditation is a one-pointed concentration meditation you may practice to cultivate mindfulness, focus, stillness, and clarity.

Gassho meditation helps us quiet our busy, preoccupied mind. When we practice *Gassho* meditation, we focus our attention on one point – the point where our middle fingers come together when our hands are placed in *Gassho* (the "prayer position"). This allows our minds to become quiet and lodged into the present moment. We can ease our restless thoughts about past events and what-ifs of the future, and silence our agendas. In this way, we learn to tame the mind, and its incessant narration, and anchor the body. When we practice *Gassho* meditation we bring stillness to the mind by focusing our attention *away* from our runaway thoughts onto the object of concentration. We practice acknowledging our thoughts, but not responding emotionally to every thought in our head.

Don't let the seeming simplicity of *Gassho* meditation fool you. Bringing our attention to what is actually happening in the present moment is challenging because it is the nature of the mind to produce one thought after another. Our difficulty comes when our thoughts spiral out on their own trajectory without us being aware that we have become the unwitting passenger on this flight. We are no longer present in the now. Ask yourself throughout the day whether you have become an unwitting passenger highjacked by your mind. The ongoing benefit of *Gassho* meditation is that we get to take our tamed mind with us wherever we go. Notice, too, how *Gassho* meditation ties in with "Just for Today," of the Reiki Precepts (Ch. 8), as we become aware that the only moment is this moment… every time.

In this *Gassho* meditation practice, the hands are placed in the "prayer position" at heart level, with the fingers pointing a bit outward, instead of pointing straight up. This evokes the expansion of our settled self *outward* to be shared with others. The bringing of the two palms together represents unifying all of the dualities of life (good/bad, I/other, better/worse, like/dislike, animate/inanimate), reminding us that, with *Gassho* meditation, we can shift our perspective from separation, division, and judgment to shared humanity. In this spaciousness, we get a taste of Usui's spiritual experience on Mt. Kurama when he expressed, *"I am within the Universe, and the Universe is within me."*

The Practice of *Gassho* Meditation:

- *Sitting in a comfortable and alert posture, place your hands together, palms facing one another at your heart level, fingertips angled slightly away from the body.*
- *Begin your hara breathing.*
- *Bringing your focus to the object of concentration – the point where your two middle fingers come together.*
- *As you breathe in and out, continuing to bring your focused attention to this object of concentration.*
- *Noticing when your thoughts distract you from this focus point of attention, and gently drawing your awareness back to the one point where the tips of your middle fingers meet.*
- *As your mind quiets, continue to focus your awareness on the point where the middle fingers meet, allowing thoughts and emotions to come, be noticed, and go, without becoming involved with them.*
- *You may notice a slight sensation where the tips of the middle fingers touch. Let your mind gently focus on that one sensation-point. You might add a bit of pressure to the point where the tips of the middle fingers touch to help sustain your focused awareness.*
- *Experiencing yourself being fully present.*

The quieter you become, the more you can hear.
– Ram Dass

Chapter 6

The Hands: Caring for Oneself with Hands-On Healing

Hands-on self-Reiki shows us how Reiki practice brings stillness into our lives, and allows us to care for ourselves in a compassionate way. This physical aspect of self-Reiki practice gets us back in touch with our bodies, deepening the mind-body connection. With self-Reiki hands-on healing, we attend to the body as we anchor the mind in the body and its physical sensations. We make no demands on the body, nor do we judge the body or its sensations.

Although some people may be familiar with Reiki as a hands-on-healing practice to care for *others*, it may be less well known that it is first and foremost a hands-on-healing practice to care for *oneself*. When we are feeling emotionally distressed or in physical pain, hands-on healing can be supportive and restorative, bringing ease and comfort to mind, body, and emotions. The self-Reiki hand placements elicit a relaxed mind-body-emotions state, shifting our nervous system from sympathetic to parasympathetic. This shift promotes optimal functioning of our body's own natural healing capacity.

Research into the physiology of touch teaches us that touch brings calm through the following pathway: By stimulating the pressure receptors in the skin, touch activates the vagus nerve which, in turn, initiates a shift into the parasympathetic nervous system. This, in turn, results in decreased heart rate and cortisol levels; improved digestion; and an increase in neurotransmitters such as serotonin which reduces the perception of pain and helps with mood (Tiffany Field 2000, 2001). When we practice self-Reiki hands-on healing we alleviate discomfort, uneasiness, and agitation. Whether we are experiencing irritability; aches and pains; upset, worry, and overwhelm; fatigue or sleeplessness, hands-on self-healing is a practical resource we can rely on for relief and as a practice for nourishing ourselves.

While the mind may wander to the future and the past, the body is always grounded in the here and now. Using the self-Reiki hand placements requires us to stop what we are doing, and get in touch with the body and bring our attention to the present moment. When we experience the connection of our touch with the body, we are drawn into inner stillness and stability; we move into feeling grounded and centered. This is in stark contrast to the frantic pace we keep in order to meet external demands. Hands-on self-Reiki practice allows us to stop and turn the focus inward. When we are in parasympathetic mode, we can tend to our distressing thoughts and emotions. Instead of pushing away our feelings or blissing-out, hands-on Reiki practice allows us to listen to our thoughts, emotions, and bodies as we care for ourselves. We feel compassion and tenderness toward ourselves. We also encourage you to practice hands-on self-healing in combination with *hara* breathing. You will find that the gentle pressure of the hands, plus the slow expansive breath, settles the nervous system so you can sit with emotions that come up, while experiencing the physiological benefits of the relaxation response.

The context in which we practice hands-on self-Reiki will vary. One of the contexts is in the moment of unease or pain. For example, if you feel a headache coming on, instead of excessively focusing on the pain, you can mindfully Pause, practice *hara* breathing, and place your hands over the area of concern with light healing touch, for 5-15 minutes, or longer if needed. [This may or may not be in combination with an over-the-counter pain reliever. As we have mentioned earlier, Reiki practice is not a replacement for medical care, and a medical doctor should always be consulted if pain persists.] Another example would be if you have a job interview in 30 minutes and are feeling anxious, you can Pause wherever you are – on the bus, on the subway, in the parking lot, or in the elevator – and practice *hara* breathing and hands-on self-Reiki to acknowledge and bring calm to anxious thoughts and feelings. These brief examples illustrate how hands-on self-Reiki can be practiced as a skill, or tool, in the very moment of distress or upset.

A second context in which we can draw on hands-on self-Reiki is as an ongoing formal, dedicated practice, at a designated time. In this case we do not need to wait for physical pain or emotional upset to occur. Instead, we practice hands-on self-Reiki as preventive health maintenance, as health creation, and/or to address any ongoing concerns we are experiencing. Building a hands-on-healing practice into our daily lives cultivates a healthy mindset with which we can approach both routine and challenging situations in skillful, balanced ways. A designated hands-on self-practice brings calm to an agitated body, encouraging healing. Keep in mind as you practice hands-on self-Reiki that healing is an *active* process for you, as healing can only come from within you. You are not the passive recipient of an external treatment; you are your own healing instrument.

Instructions for a Formal, Dedicated Practice of Hands-On Self-Reiki

- Throughout this practice of hands-on self-Reiki, sense into the contact points between your hands and your body.
- Set aside a space and time that is comfortable for you.
- Landing here now, knowing you belong to this moment, and this moment belongs to you.
- Practice *hara* breathing to stabilize and settle mind and body.
- Silently stating the intent that you will begin hands-on healing to care for yourself in a compassionate way.

The Self-Reiki Hand Placements

Hold each placement 3-5 minutes, or more, as desired, and continue *hara* breathing:

Hand Placements on the Head

Placing your hands comfortably on the crown of your head. (Comfort hint: If you are seated and there is a table in front of you, consider resting your elbows on the table to support your arms, instead of raising your arms above shoulder level.)

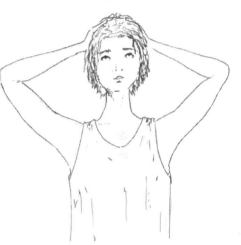

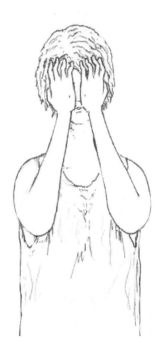

Cupping your hands gently over the front of your face, resting your fingertips on the hairline and the heel of your hands on the lower face. (Comfort hint: If you are seated, rest your arms on your chest for support.)

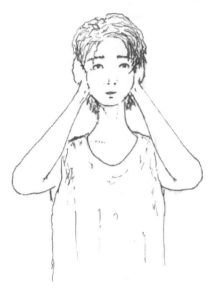

Bringing your hands to the sides of your head, gently covering the ears and jaw line. (Comfort hint: If you are seated, experiment with what is more comfortable for you; orienting your elbows forward versus downward.)

Moving the hands to the back of the head, with one hand covering the occipital ridge (just above the neck) and the other hand just above the lower hand. See diagram for an alternative as well, finding the one most comfortable for you. (Comfort hint: If you are seated, lean back into the chair to support yourself.)

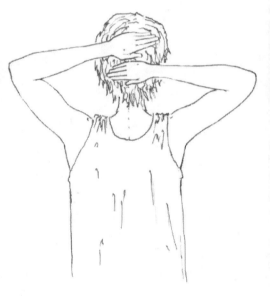

Hand Placements on the Neck, Chest, and Torso

Bringing your hands to the front of your body and place the hands over the throat. See diagrams for two options for this throat hand placement. Please find the one that is most comfortable for you.

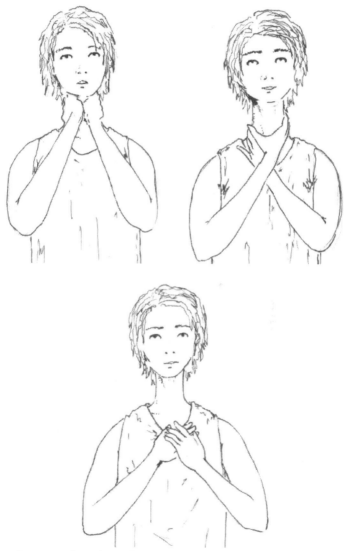

Lowering your hands to the upper chest, at approximately heart level. Usually your hands will overlap each other in the center of the upper chest. Alternatively, it may feel more natural to you to place your hands across the upper chest with the fingertips meeting at the midline of the body.

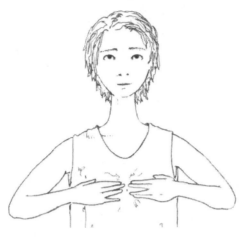

Lowering your hands once again and place hands over the mid-chest, with fingers meeting at the midline of the body.

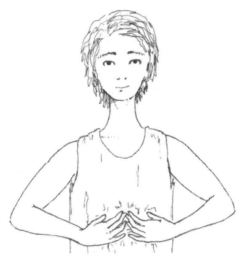

Lowering the hands to the upper abdomen, just under the ribcage; typically your left hand will be approximately where the stomach, spleen, and pancreas are located, and the right hand approximately where the liver is located.

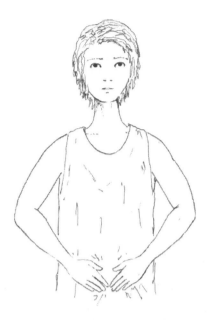

Lowering the hands to the area of the middle abdomen.

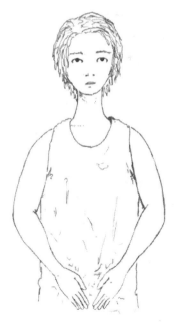

Lowering the hands a little further to the area of the lower abdomen.

You may choose to place the hands on any joints of the body you can comfortably reach (upper body: shoulders and elbows; lower body: hips, knees, and ankles).

If it is comfortable for you, you can "sandwich" each foot between your hands.

While the self-Reiki hand placement protocol offers a reassuring guideline for self-practice, it is by no means rigid. For example, if you are feeling irritated or agitated, you may discover there is a specific area of the body on which placing your hands, for 5-15 minutes, or longer, will bring the most comfort and help you settle. This shows that your *own* direct experience is the best guide, allowing you to tailor hands-on self-healing to your own needs, as you adapt the hand placements for yourself.

"Reiki Relief Remedy": Special Hand Placement for Calm

Sometimes our hectic days scatter and drain us, on other days we may experience intense feelings of panic and fear, and on

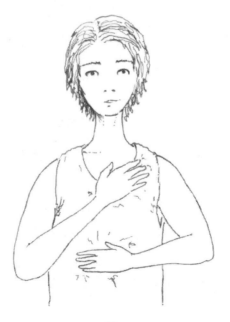

yet other days we are aware of persistent agitation or worry gnawing at us. The "Reiki Relief Remedy" hand placement helps us traverse the landscape of these feelings, and lessen our distress. For example, we may notice troubling thoughts gripping us, disturbing our composure; this is the perfect time for "Reiki Relief Remedy" to the rescue! The authors find themselves using this go-to hand placement frequently throughout their days to settle and calm an agitated body and mind. We acknowledge that this practice may not *change* distressing *external* circumstances, but it *can* change how we *relate* to these circumstances.

- *Standing, sitting, or lying down, place one hand comfortably on the upper chest and the other hand comfortably on the abdomen just below the sternum where the ribs separate (solar plexus).*
- *At the same time, practice hara breathing to gain further benefit of down-regulating the nervous system.*
- *With gentle pressure of hands on the body, remain in this calming position for as long as you feel is right for you. Feel the connection between the palms of your hands and your body. Appreciate what you can do on your own to settle your body and mind.*

Chapter 7

The Centers of Awareness: The 3 Diamonds of *Ki*

Body Like the Mountain, Mind Like the Sky, Heart Like the Ocean
– Dogen Zenji (1200-1253)

The teaching by Dogen Zenji, "Body like a Mountain, Mind like the Sky, Heart like the Ocean," introduces us to the Japanese concept of the 3 Diamonds of *Ki*. *Ki* can be thought of as "the energy that sustains and nourishes all life," and we can all cultivate *ki* with Reiki self-practices that strengthen and support our self-awareness. It is helpful to understand the 3 Diamonds of *Ki* as inner resources of awareness of (1) our body, (2) our mind, and (3) our heart (Wilberg 2003: x-xii). When we become aware of our body like a mountain we claim the solid, strong, rooted qualities within ourselves. When we become aware of our mind like the sky, we get in touch with our qualities of open-mindedness, spaciousness, and expansiveness. When we become aware of our heart like the ocean, we reach for our inner qualities of connection, inter-being, compassion, and loving expression.

Let's look at each of the 3 Diamonds of *Ki* and their associated practices.

Earth *Ki* ~ Body Like a Mountain

Mindfulness of Body focuses our awareness on the qualities of Earth *Ki* within us and the focus is the *Hara*: Here we bring our attention to our solid base or foundation. When we rest our mind on the *hara* and the qualities of Earth *Ki* within us, we nurture a sense of being solid, stable, focused and grounded. When we experience these sensations we are like a solid mountain. From this center of awareness we can hold our own when storms of turmoil rage around us, and when provocations come at us. We drop anchor within ourselves. From this solid foundation, we can manage our fears and uncertainties with greater resilience so our foundation is less likely to split apart. When we have *hara* awareness, there is always access to a sustainable source of strength and courage whenever needed. The inner attitude that *hara* awareness brings allows us to improve our ability to cope with both everyday tasks and sudden emergencies with greater ease because we are stable and solid.

This solidity is not only confined to the *hara*. Earth *Ki* brings stability to the mind as well, so our mind is settled and available.

We invite you to take a moment right now to experience your body like a mountain with this Mindfulness of Body meditation:

Practice of Mindfulness of Body/Hara/Earth *Ki* Meditation:

1. *Closing your eyes if comfortable, place your hands restfully on your hara space (3 finger-widths below your naval).*
2. *Bringing your awareness to your abdomen.*
3. *Focusing on the hara, and feel it as a space of solidity and strength.*
4. *Breathing in through your nose, feel yourself breathing into that inner space; the surface of your abdomen rising and expanding as you breathe in a refreshing breath. Focusing on how the in-breath descends into the hara space.*
5. *As you breathe out through your nose or mouth, allow and notice how your breath expands gently out into your surroundings.*
6. *Experiencing the hara as an inner sanctuary in which you can settle and rest within yourself.*
7. *Sensing a still-point of silence in the inner space of your abdomen (Wilberg 2003: 136).*
8. *Experiencing yourself listening into this still-point of silence*

(Wilberg 2003: 136).

9. Experiencing your exhalations as an out-breath of expansive awareness of the qualities of Earth Ki within yourself: feeling settled and solid; grounded and composed.

10. Like the Earth, this is your inner Earth Ki – the qualities of Earth Ki sustain and anchor you, even when the mind is turbulent, and the spirit feels drained.

11. Feeling yourself looking out at the world from this center of awareness in the hara.

12. Reflecting for a moment within yourself: What is your perspective and way of experiencing the world from this center of awareness of Earth Ki?

Let's now see what is happening in the two other centers of awareness.

Sky *Ki* ~ Mind Like the Sky

Mindfulness of Mind focuses our awareness on the qualities of Sky *Ki* within us and the focus is the head: Here we bring attention to our mind being awake, alert, and spacious. In this center of awareness we experience our mind as vast, clear, and open like the sky. We acknowledge things as they are, instead of leaping to judge them. We can recognize our thoughts with sympathy so we can be gently open to our own ups and downs. To avoid feeling spacey, though, we anchor the mind in the qualities of Earth *Ki*. We all know that when the mind spins out on a runaway train, it's hard to connect with our hearts, our *hara*, let alone with one another. When we experience balance between Sky *Ki* and Earth *Ki* we are less caught up with, and less driven by, plans, judgments, expectations, and regrets. Mindfulness of Sky *Ki* helps us claim a wider perspective, broad-mindedness, and wisdom.

Vast and spacious as the sky, this is our mind without the dualistic labeling. When we label and get attached to dualistic thoughts our mind becomes cluttered, boxed in, and narrow. When we can naturally experience this openness of mind without effort this is the process. Having the ability to sustain and maintain this vastness of mind, this spaciousness of mind and clarity of mind in all situations in life is called Perfect Happiness.
– KM Chukdong

Practice of Sky *Ki* Meditation:

1. *Closing your eyes if comfortable, place your hands restfully anywhere on the head, including the face.*
2. *Becoming aware of your head.*
3. *Sensing a center of awareness in this space.*
4. *Feeling your mind as alert, awake, clear, and steady, and from these qualities, feeling your mind as vast and spacious, like the sky.*
5. *Inhaling a refreshing Ki-filled breath through your nose.*
6. *Exhaling slowly, sensing you are reaching forward into the space in front and around you from the center of awareness in your head (Wilberg 2003: 133).*
7. *Reflecting for a moment within yourself: What is your perspective and way of knowing of the world from this center of awareness of spacious Sky Ki?*

Heart *Ki* ~ Heart Like the Ocean

Mindfulness of Heart focuses our awareness on the qualities of Heart *Ki* within us and the focus is the center of the chest: Here we bring attention to our hearts like the ocean. We may stand on a beach counting each wave as it crashes, 1, 2, 3, 4. But each wave, seemingly solitary, is connected to every other wave. And all of the waves are connected to the ocean as a whole. Each ocean connected to every other ocean. We feel connected, like waves in the ocean, to our common humanity and inter-being with all things. We extend our humanity with gentleness, loving-kindness, tenderness, and generosity. The basic quality of Heart *Ki* is spaciousness, which is timeless and limitless; eternal. We feel expansive, without limits or constriction. We feel deep caring and warmth for others, knowing that their suffering is not different from our own. When we open our hearts, we experience our common humanity. We are not so separated from others by our likes and dislikes, but extend our heart beyond these likes and dislikes. We open our hearts and find we can experience a loving, expansive relationship with all things. Mindfulness of Heart is what "YES" feels like – open, spacious, enhancing your spirit and vitality. When we feel a sense of inter-being with all things, we experience participation consciousness.

Humans have evolved to give and receive care and nurturing. Even more, we evolved *to feel good* when we connect with others with compassion and lovingkindness – an open heart like the ocean. When we open our hearts and share our hearts with others we have nothing to hide; no suit of armor. From the center of awareness of Heart *Ki*, we can expand our vision and give fearlessly to others, strengthening ourselves to carry out social justice work. Returning to the "heart of things" is the point of balance reached by harmonizing body, mind, and heart. Even with pain and struggle in life, we see people show their deepest humanity, and we too become part of that whole when we say "yes" and open the heart like the ocean.

When asked, "How are we to treat others?"
Ramana Maharshi replied, "There are no others."

Practice of Heart *Ki* Meditation:

1.   *Closing your eyes if comfortable, rest the hands gently over the center of the chest.*

2. *Bringing your awareness into the heart space in the center of your chest.*

3. *Sensing this space as an inner sanctuary.*

4. *Breathing in and sense your chest expanding and filling with Ki. Exhale and expand that refreshed Ki-filled breath out into the space around you.*

5. *Slowly opening your eyes and bringing your attention to your surroundings, including any people that may be present.*

6. *Feeling yourself aware of everything that fills the space around you with the qualities of appreciation and thankfulness based in Heart Ki.*

7. *Feeling yourself absorbing awareness and appreciation of your surroundings through your heart.*

8. *As you exhale, sensing your heart opening and expanding from this center of awareness of Heart Ki.*

9. *Feeling yourself experiencing and perceiving the world from this center of awareness; from this inner Heart Ki resource found within.*

10. *Reflecting for a moment within yourself: What is your awareness of the world from this center of awareness of Heart Ki?*

With 3 Diamonds of *Ki* practice we can become mindful of our body and of the state of our *kokoro,* so we can live consciously aware and awake to all possibilities, while being grounded and settled. When we bring together Earth *Ki* and Sky *Ki*, we can express Heart *Ki* genuinely and naturally, and we can live intentionally.

Anecdote: Here is a real-life anecdote to illustrate what is possible for us and others when we make a conscious effort to stay anchored, yet open-minded and open-hearted in everyday situations: *Graciella had recently embarked on a solid small business venture, and everything was falling into place. It was time for Graciella* to set up a way for her customers to make payments online through her website. She moved forward with a company, but was experiencing difficulties, so she called the Customer Service Department. As someone who already brought Reiki practice into her life, Graciella chose to do some hara breathing during the long wait time on the phone. When it was her turn, she described her predicament to the CSR, at which time the CSR transferred her to someone else. After another 10 minute wait on hold, accompanied by ever more needed hara breathing, Graciella got on line with a new CSR, assuming this individual had already been updated on her situation. Alas, no, that was not the case, and Graciella found herself feeling the energy of impatience and aggravation rise in her body. And, at that moment, she was put on hold again. Having become familiar with herself and her reactions, Graciella knew she was facing a choice: allow her reactions to control her, or invite into this moment the Reiki 3 Diamonds of Ki practice. Beginning with mindfulness of body, Graciella focused awareness on her hara and the qualities of being solid and settled like a mountain. In that moment she could trust herself to hang in there and deal with things. But Graciella wanted to do more than "deal with" things, so she took another moment to experience mindfulness of mind, visualizing and feeling her mind as vast and open as the sky. She felt an expansive outlook and a perspective that allowed her to be aware of the situation with less reactivity. With mindfulness of heart, Graciella connected with her heart being like the ocean, she felt she could be receptive to whatever and whomever she would encounter. When the CSR came back to the phone, Graciella felt both refreshed and anchored and found she could access a calm and tender awareness within herself. And, even better, she reclaimed her lively sense of humor and not only got her problem solved, but was able to bring some levity to the conversation. She felt good about moving forward with this company and ever more committed to her small business... and her Reiki self-practice. This anecdote illustrates how the 3 Diamonds of Ki meditative practice is beneficial and practical in everyday situations. When we face aggravation we can utilize the 3 Diamonds of *Ki* meditation to claim awareness from all 3 centers of awareness.

Chapter 8

The Compass: The 5 Reiki Precepts

Inviting Happiness through many blessings; the spiritual medicine
for all ills...
Just for today...
Do not fuel anger
Do not fuel worry
Practice Gratitude
Live Honestly
Show Compassion to all beings

Popularly, the system of Reiki is often thought of as being limited to hands-on healing, but the 5 Reiki Precepts, as well as the breathing practice and meditations introduced earlier, are vital resources for healing the deepest parts of ourselves. The 5 Reiki Precepts offer us a compass along a path toward mindfulness, emotional freedom, resilience and spiritual growth. The Reiki Precepts are the heart of the system of Reiki and are all about cultivating self-awareness of our heart/mind-state and living in accord with our most meaningful values. By engaging with the Precepts we can relate kindly to our experiences of anger, worry, and fear, and cultivate a consciousness of gratitude, integrity, and compassion. A commitment to living in accord with the five Reiki Precepts brings a healthy heart-mind (*kokoro*), which in turn supports the body. When we embody the Precepts, we can more kindly relate to the habits of mind such as anger, worry, fear, impatience, and resentment. We can reclaim qualities we already have within ourselves such as courage, gratitude, compassion, and patience. In this way we can live authentically, in accord with our deepest values. Living in alignment with the Precepts frees us to claim the human potential already within us. It is important to remember that the Precepts are not meant to be used as a means to judge or reject any part of ourselves or others, rather the Precepts describe ways of being that are within our reach.

Connecting with the Reiki Precepts throughout the day helps us become aware of the habitual thoughts and patterns of behavior that bring us to anger and worry. So day by day we become mindful of the conditionings in ourselves, and why we think, feel and act the way we do. Working with the 5 Precepts may bring insight into those things that are not yet healed in ourselves, and with this awareness, we may better be able to free ourselves of the conditionings that cause our suffering. With this sense of freedom, we are better able to see areas of suffering around us, and respond to the needs of others with compassion and caring words and actions.

We want to share with you the analogy of the knot. Each time a person or circumstance in our lives disappoints or frightens us, a knot of fear, worry, anxiety, or anger is tightened within us. Without tools and practices to loosen and untangle the knot, it grows tighter and tighter around each painful experience. Mindfulness of the Precepts helps us untangle the knots, freeing our *kokoro* (heart-mind). Instead of suppressing and fighting anger, worry, and fear, we can learn important lessons from these mind-states and experiences, and disentangle the knots. With the Precepts we are observing our internal state: maybe we notice defensiveness or the need to be right; maybe we become aware of our impatience, or our constant judgment and criticism of others; maybe we become aware of our thirst for approval. The Precepts remind us to be mindful and aware of our reactivity, inviting in more gentleness, acceptance, humility, and ease. These ways of being are an antidote to resisting and fighting our own experiences. This is the foundation of real healing, as our own thoughts and feelings about our experiences create the terrain for suffering... or for freedom. Observing ourselves in light of the Precepts expands outward into our daily lives as we extend the spirit of the Precepts – living with Precepts awareness – beyond ourselves.

Our daily life is where the Precepts are put into practice.

Anecdote: Here is an instructive anecdote from a Reiki practitioner, recorded verbatim, that exemplifies that our daily life is where the Precepts are put into practice: *"Who here has ever worked in retail?! I am not kidding when I share with you that, at the end of the day, when we locked the door and put out the 'Closed' sign, we would gather in a huddle and yell, 'People drive us nuts!' The pressure of pleasing challenging customers took its toll on our attitude and mood. Following several months of self-Reiki practice, including a commitment to the Precepts, I surprised myself by speaking with kindness to even the most challenging customers even when I felt judgment bubbling up. Refraining from participating in hurtful speech, and bringing kindness instead, became its own reward as I felt emotionally free, comfortable, and at ease. With this kindness, the customers were also more at ease. I would go so far as to say, the Precepts were indeed the key to inviting happiness into my life and my workplace."*

Let's look at the impact each of these Precepts can have in our lives.

Just for today...
Do not fuel anger
Do not fuel worry
Practice Gratitude
Live Honestly
Show Compassion to all beings

Just for Today

This is a gentle and practical reminder to focus on the present moment. The present moment is the only time we have to be mindful of what thoughts, feelings, and actions are happening, and from there we can make a choice to speak and act from a calmer, more settled, compassionate self. And isn't it true that *every* moment *is this* moment. We can enact the Precepts only in the now. Each moment is all that we have. Each moment brings us a choice of what to pay attention to. Each moment brings a choice of how we will respond and what we will say and do. Each moment brings a choice of self-imprisonment or of freedom. A "Just for Today" consciousness means we notice our reactions with awareness and acknowledgement, without resistance. *Just for Today* reminds us that moment by moment we can live our lives in accord with the Precepts so we can live peacefully with ourselves and others.

The structure of the 5 Reiki Precepts is significant because the *first two* Precepts (Do Not Fuel Anger; Do Not Fuel Worry) teach us that anger, worry, and fear bring *separation* and distance from others. While the *last three* Precepts (Practice Gratitude, Live Honestly, Show Compassion to all Beings) teach us that we can create *connection and closeness* with others by living honestly, practicing gratitude, and showing compassion.

1st Precept ~ Do Not Fuel Anger

What is anger? It is an intense, but natural, emotion, built into all mammals, in response to threats directed at us. Anger also results when things in our lives are not playing out the way we want them to, when we don't feel listened to or understood, and when our needs aren't being met. When people and circumstances are not what we want them to be, we can easily feel anger. Anger isn't just one thing: we may experience anger as feelings of impatience, irritation, frustration, hurt, sadness, helplessness, lack of control, or disappointment. When we pay attention to these feelings, they can teach us a lot about ourselves, yet they can also constrict us and tie us up in knots. In fact, the Japanese character for anger means "slave to our heart-mind" (*kokoro*) (Pearson 2018: 95). When we lack self-awareness of our own angry feelings, we are the source of *our own* enslavement. Reiki self-practice with the first Precept, "Do Not Fuel Anger," teaches us that when we are mindful of our anger, we can loosen the knot of habitual anger.

It is likely that, for most of us, anger comes from an understandable fear of the uncertainty and fragility of life from which we naturally want to protect ourselves. So we are not advocates of condemning, shaming, or suppressing the emotion of anger. In fact, all emotions are a dimension of our beings. Rather, we encourage practice of the mindful Pause (Ch. 4) and *hara* breathing (Ch. 3) to *relate to* the emotional experience – the what, when, and why of our anger. Let's remember, the human experience is wide and broad, and includes love, compassion, and gratitude, as well as anger and fear.

Let's recognize that we may hesitate to acknowledge anger in ourselves.

Nonetheless, it *is* part of the human experience to feel frustration, irritation, and anger when we don't get what we want, when our expectations are not met, and when we feel threatened.

So even though we may have been told *not* to get angry, it is quite natural to feel anger when things are not going the way we want and troubling things happen that are beyond our control. Of course, there is a difference between *having* an angry feeling and *acting* on that anger.

It's common to *feel* anger in the mind-body. Anger is a state of mind; an emotional experience, and we feel it in the body; but anger in itself is not harmful *action*. But when we *fuel* that anger, we can cause harm to self and others with our words and actions. While it may be uncomfortable and unpleasant to acknowledge

The Compass: The 5 Reiki Precepts

our anger, the more we listen to ourselves, the more we can accept our anger without judgment as one part of what we are in our human experience.

So how do we *not* fuel anger? Whenever we're feeling frustrated or angry, instead of going into our old patterns of thinking, speaking, and acting, we can try another, more intentional, way. In other words, we may *notice* and *acknowledge* angry feelings moment by moment, but we do not have to *live* in anger or fuel anger. Instead, we can Pause in stillness to notice and acknowledge we are, in fact, experiencing the emotion of anger. Second, we can support ourselves with hands-on Reiki practice (Ch. 6) and/or *hara* breathing (Ch. 3) as we tune into the bodily sensations of our anger, hurt, and fear. We may notice tightness in the chest, for example. And, then, over time, we become more and more aware of the signs of annoyance and frustration as they bubble up in our bodies and minds. Third, the key is to *stay with* these feelings and sensations, even when doing so feels uncomfortable. Fourth, see that by sensing the solidity of the *hara*, we can hang in there with any pain and discomfort that the anger brings out in us without feeding or fueling the anger. We see that it's actually okay to experience ourselves as we are in any given moment. Fifth, when we stay with the angry feelings for a bit, but do not escalate or act on them, we can better see our anger as information about what is happening in our mind-body. In this way we are not the source of our own self-enslavement. Our anger can indicate to us something that may need attention, something essential about our mind-body, or about the external situation, that we actually need to be aware of in order to feel whole.

It is pretty much guaranteed that we will feel better when we practice self-awareness of emotion and self-control of action, instead of operating on reactive auto-pilot. For example, imagine that someone is tailgating you on the highway. If you leap to act on angry feelings, you could cause an accident. But

The Compass: The 5 Reiki Precepts

there is another possibility: when you pause and notice your anger and fear, you don't have to *fuel* them. You can choose a different way of responding that reaches beyond your habitual reaction of aggravation and anger. You don't have to be trapped by your knee-jerk reactions. Even in heated and difficult moments, if our minds are calmer and clearer we can regulate our emotions and respond in more productive, skillful ways. By taking a pause and regulating ourselves, we can almost neutralize the emotional impact an event otherwise may have caused. This brings to mind the story told in Chapter 4 about the Zen teacher who taught that the most important life lesson is about responding appropriately.

Not *living* in anger is critical to our physical well-being. We know that holding onto anger can be harmful to our health. Anger can poison our bodies and souls. We can feel this in our own bodies, as anger puts us out of balance. Indeed, anger is the antithesis of balance. In Chapter 2, we introduced you to the Stress Response which results in the wear and tear of all the systems of the body. Living in anger can harm our immune system, whereas a settled mind-body strengthens it. Furthermore, living in anger can ignite inflammatory processes in the body, whereas emotional steadiness can reduce inflammation.

We also might find ourselves around angry people. How do we not let *their* anger disturb *our* equilibrium? The other person may be living in anger, but we do not have to live there *with* them. When we bring awareness to the situation, we can realize that the other person's anger is coming from *their* own place of distress, and may actually have nothing to do with us. With this realization, we are then free from taking responsibility for the angry feelings of others, when it is not ours to take. Think of how emotionally freeing that is!

The question often arises, is there ever *useful* anger? We think so. We can see brutality all around us: bullying; sexual harassment; domestic violence; incivility; social media misuse;

political indecency; racial injustice. Wherever we find imbalances of power and maldistribution of resources, we find inhumanity. When we notice the anger that arises within us in response to this heartlessness, we can address that anger by taking productive action to redress injustice. Rather than seething in anger, we can transform and mobilize that anger to take wise action to address societal ills [More on this is Chapter 11].

As described in Chapters 3 and 4 on *hara* breathing and the mindful Pause, we can equip ourselves with the skills to notice and acknowledge our angry feelings and then regulate our reactions. We can use our Reiki mind-body skills to modulate our potentially harmful reactions, creating a new mindset, being open to possibilities, and freeing ourselves from the entanglement and enslavement of both our own minds, as well as of provocative situations.

> *I will practice mindful breathing and walking to recognize and look deeply into my anger... I will speak and listen in such a way as to help myself and the other person to transform suffering and to see the way out of difficult situations.*
> – Thich Nhat Hanh

Contemplation Exercise to Engage with the 1st Precept ~ *Do Not Fuel Anger*

Our anger may contain a wealth of information, especially about where there is fear and threat for us; where we feel vulnerable, afraid, and in need of self-protection. So it is helpful to see our anger as a teacher that can help us become more familiar with ourselves. When unaddressed, anger does not simply disappear; rather, it may become internalized and drain us, or may become externalized as rage.

Ask yourself with curiosity, care and kindness:

When am I most angry?

What circumstances and interactions trigger angry reactions in
me?
Who am I without fueling this anger?
What do I bring into my life without fueling this anger?
What do I bring into the world without fueling this anger?

Contemplate:

When I am mindful of feelings of anger, I can take care of, and
soften, my feelings of anger.
When I take care of my feelings of anger, I can gain insight into
what is behind that anger.
When I notice anger arise within me, I do not have to fuel it.

Anecdote: When we are unexpectedly betrayed by a person
whom we thought we could trust, we can feel enormous shock,
disappointment, hurt, and anger. *A hard-working employee, James,
loyal to his boss and coworkers, is primed for a promotion. James'
boss had told him that he would be the next in line for the position.
Upon arriving to work one day, James overheard his coworkers talking
about another person who was to fill the position instead. James felt
shocked and betrayed, and his initial impulse was to angrily confront
his boss. Seething with rage, James walks toward his boss' office,
feeling his face get red, his heart pounding. He is about to let loose
with an angry outburst. On that short walk down the corridor, James
becomes aware of the intensity of the anger in his body.* James is able
to take a Mindful Pause and shift both his consciousness and
his physiology into a calmer, settled state because he has been
working with Reiki practices, including the Precepts. He did not
fuel his anger, he softened his anger, thereby giving himself time
and space to think about how he could approach the situation in
a skillful manner.

2nd Precept ~ Do Not Fuel Worry

Let's uncover worry. The tendency to worry is to some extent built into the human experience so we can be alert to potential dangers and problems and prepare ourselves accordingly. What can be harmful, though, is when worry and anxious thoughts about the uncertainties of life dominate our lives and cause us suffering and erode our resilience. We acknowledge, and sympathize with, the devastating circumstances in many of our lives in which worry may become disabling. It is interesting to note that the Japanese word for worry has two characters which can be translated as "distribute the heart's wholeness" (Pearson 2018: 97). And we do, in fact, experience worry as being broken, shattered, and as having a hole in our center. When we are overcome with worry, we have allowed our power, intactness, and peace to literally disperse or drain from our being. Interestingly, in English, the word worry can be traced back to the word "strangled." When we are strangled with worry, we are constricted and immobilized. Both cultures recognize that worry drains and paralyzes us.

It can be fear-provoking and overwhelming to realize that many life circumstances are completely out of our control. How do we live with that truth of life's fragility? How do we navigate all of the uncertainties of life? We first have to become aware that the potential for fear and worry naturally lie within us, and these emotions can make us feel overwhelmed and miserable, and cause unnecessary suffering. In his teachings, Elisha Goldstein reminds us that there is no actual "cure" for worry. With Reiki self-practice, though, we can move into new ways to relate to, and be with, the intense discomfort of worry, and invite in a sense of balance and perspective. One of the benefits we can experience with Reiki practice is awareness that, although we cannot control external conditions, we can influence our inner state. Ruminating on our worries serves no useful purpose; it just brings suffering. This is when we need a deliberate mindful pause to cause an effect within us. The system of Reiki provides us with specific practices, introduced in this book, that allow us to experience a softening of the worry that afflicts us. We discover that we do not have to live in worry, or fuel the worry that may arise. When we become aware of uneasy, worried feelings, our self-Reiki skills can help us be with these feelings without being controlled and strangled by them. Practicing with this Precept helps us manage the vicious cycle of distressing worried and anxious thinking that can devastate us – body, mind, and spirit.

Worry can also burden and strangle those about whom we worry. Our intense feelings of worry encumber others, leaving them with increased worry and anxiety, eventually eroding the relationship. Fear and worry are contagious! By working with this Precept over time, not only do we free ourselves from suffering, but we free others as well.

One of the most valuable teachings to be aware of is that, similar to anger, behind worry is often fear. When we are consumed by chronic worry and fear we habitually interpret the world through that lens. Unfortunately, this creates separation and distance from everything and everyone. A mindset of worry distances us from those about whom we worry, even when we rationalize our worry as concern for their best interest. When we worry, we may think we are being helpful and connected, however, we may actually be trying to control the situation to assuage our own fears, and protect ourselves from the feelings of having no control. If, for example, I am gripped by worry about a loved one's whereabouts, it may appear that I am caring and connected, when in fact I am self-absorbed and preoccupied by my own distress and my own need to control a situation over which I really have no control. At times like this choosing to practice Reiki mind-body skills allows us to disengage from the grip of our own mind which is habituated to worry and fear. It is inevitable that we experience some worry and fear, however, self-Reiki practice strengthens us to hold these strong emotions without having them define and constrict us. Further, we may gain insight into our worry and fear, figuring out what is behind them, thereby reducing their hold on us. When we are less self-absorbed with our worry, we are free to experience genuine closeness and connection with others.

Although it may seem like it is the people and circumstances around us that create our emotional response of worry, it is actually us. We actually perpetuate our worry by exercising the harmful "muscle" of worry and fear. And the more often we find ourselves in this worried, fearful state, the more we are activating and exercising the part of us that reacts with worry and fear. It is like using a muscle over and over; it becomes bigger. But there is something we can do as an antidote to the cycle of worry and fear, allowing us to free ourselves from rumination and separation. The 2nd Precept, along with the Reiki mind-body practices introduced in this book, gives us a way to exercise a new, healthful "muscle": the muscle of self-awareness of our worry mind-state. Strengthening this muscle of self-awareness will reduce the emotional charge and stranglehold of worry and fear.

One of the traps we can fall into is letting our worry take on a life of its own, overwhelming us with the misperception that this is all we are. Sometimes we have to agree to let the worry and fear be there, but we don't have to let them define us. We can just accept that they are *one part* of us but not our whole identity. What can we do?! With ongoing Reiki self-practice, and commitment to our own well-being, we can hold and care for our worried, fearful feelings without being strangled by them. We all want to be available and open... and we can. When we do not fuel worry we can create an inner terrain where we can flourish and connect to others with an open heart.

Who is your enemy? Mind is your enemy.
No one can harm you more than a mind untrained.

Who is your friend? Mind is your friend.
Nothing can help you more than a trained mind.
– The Buddha

Anecdote: If you are anything like Anna, you have experienced paralyzing worry about a child. *Once Anna's children were able to have some independence, such as riding their bikes to the local store at age 10, Anna's worry intensified as she felt no control to protect them: Would someone snatch them? Would they get hit by a car? Would they fall and get injured? The ultimate worry was whether the children would return safely home; a situation over which Anna had no control. After bikes, it was cars, and Anna's worry escalated in step with the level of danger and distance. When we are witness to Anna's experience of worry, we see she was clearly suffering and in distress. She could feel the worry as symptoms in her body – head spinning, shortness of breath, heart racing, stomach churning. The worry did not result only in Anna's physical and emotional pain; her worry also burdened her children. The kids were aware of their mother's constant worry, which caused them to feel suffocated and retreat. This is the exact opposite of what Anna truly wanted in her relationship with her children. When Anna discovered Reiki practice, and the 2nd Precept, she learned that she had to own her worry; that worry lived inside of her and was not really caused by bike rides and driver's licenses. Anna discovered that she was, in fact, burdening her children with her need for control. This process of hard-won self-awareness of her worry, and the internal and external harm it caused, allowed Anna to rewrite the "worry script." She said to herself, "The process stops here; I am not going to pass this suffering to my children any longer."* Although it took time for Anna to move into a state of greater ease, with ongoing self-Reiki practice she could feel the grip of worry release over time. It is clear from this example that engaging with this Precept, Do Not Fuel Worry, can be life-changing, bringing emotional freedom and personal growth to all sides of a relationship.

Contemplation Exercise to Engage with the 2nd Precept ~ *Do Not Fuel Worry*

Our worry contains a wealth of information, especially about where there is fear, threat, and a lack of control leaving us feeling helpless and powerless. When unaddressed, worry does not disappear; rather, worry may drain the life right out of us, or fill our days with miserable, frantic overwhelm.

Ask yourself with curiosity, care and kindness:

> *When am I most worried?*
> *What are the circumstances that trigger worried feelings in me?*
> *Who am I without being gripped by worry?*
> *What do I bring into my life without fueling worry?*
> *What do I bring into the world without being gripped by worry?*

Contemplate:

> *When I am mindful of feelings of worry, I can take care of my feelings of worry.*
> *When I take care of my feelings of worry, I can gain insight into what is behind that worry.*
> *When I notice worry arise within me, I do not have to fuel it. By not fueling the worry, I trust myself to sit with my fearful feelings about the things that I cannot control... and be alright.*

As we noted earlier, the structure of the 5 Reiki Precepts is significant because the first two (Do Not Fuel Anger; Do Not Fuel Worry) are all about how we create *separation* and *distance* from self and others with our unchecked anger, worry and fear. With self-Reiki practice, we can gradually move into overcoming the anger, worry, and fear that fuel this separation and distance from others. By contrast, the last three Precepts (Practice Gratitude, Living Honestly, Show Compassion to all Beings), which we introduce next, are about how we can "open out" to create connection and closeness with others.

3rd *Precept ~ Practice Gratitude*

Gratitude lies in the center of the 5 Precepts because it is pivotal to our commitment to *shin shin kaizen* (ongoing self-development). The Precept, Practice Gratitude, is located after the Precepts, Do Not Fuel Anger and Do Not Fuel Worry, for a reason. "Practice Gratitude" reminds us that when we *don't* carry anger and worry, we have more space to focus on the things that really carry deep meaning. We often think that gratitude is about making a list of all the things for which we are grateful. Although this is a beneficial practice, Mikao Usui, the founder of the system of Reiki, likely had more in mind when reflecting on Gratitude. This Precept is more about a *state of being* than it is about composing a list of things we are grateful for. By cultivating a *mindset* of gratitude we become aware of that which is fulfilling in our lives and in the world. This can really vitalize and uplift us! When we feel receptive in this way, we are more available and responsive to people and situations. The emotion of gratitude inspires us to pay it forward, feel part of a network of reciprocity, and experience real participation consciousness and spiritual expression.

This is, however, not such an easy task. Gratitude is not just a sentimental notion; gratitude is active, requiring practice. Practicing gratitude can be easy when our lives are sailing along smoothly.

But when we are facing hardship, gripped by anger or worry, and feeling vulnerable, it may be impossible to even have the notion of practicing gratitude. In order to cope with hardships we tend to build a protective barrier around ourselves for fear of letting more hurt in. While this self-protective coping response is natural, it comes with a down-side: our world constricts around us. While we may feel protected from allowing further hurt in, at the same time we may be missing sources of nourishment, growth, and fulfillment that may be hidden from view. Because we all face hardship and uncertainty, and self-protection is a natural reaction, we assert that gratitude is something to be *practiced* as much as it is an outlook.

You may be wondering by now, how does one actually *practice* gratitude? The word practice reminds us that gratitude is not only an attitude; it requires deliberate awareness and follow-through. The good things we experience may be very small, and if we are not mindful we will miss them completely. When we can practice bringing our attention to our surroundings – such as being the recipient of an unexpected kindness, or the appearance of a favorite animal on our path – we may be able to touch a sense of appreciation. This *is* the experience of practicing gratitude; it is openness to awe. Imagine yourself pausing with a mindset of thankfulness-filled awe: wouldn't the body feel relaxed and at ease, but also vitalized, as you rest your consciousness on that which evokes your sense of awe and gratitude? As discussed in Chapter 2, when our body feels relaxed and at ease, we elicit the parasympathetic nervous system, facilitating a healing state. At the same time, this experience of appreciation encourages a sense of spaciousness, aliveness, and spiritual vitality in which we are moved beyond the confines of the self. You know that feeling when your heart opens and you feel less constricted and more connected? This is the feeling of gratitude. Although approaching our lives with gratitude does not magically take our problems away, it certainly can change the mindset we live in day-to-day.

Two Japanese concepts further elucidate the feeling of thankfulness-filled awe and awareness of interconnection. *Jiriki* means "self-power," and refers to *our own* efforts. *Tariki* means "other power," and refers to knowing that we cannot accomplish anything apart from others. It is awareness of *tariki* that brings gratitude out from within. With *tariki* we notice our interdependence with all things and feel appreciation for all that is beyond ourselves. Life can become ever more expansive when we acknowledge the significance of interdependence with all things. Take something as simple as a cotton shirt you wear – we can appreciate the cotton plant, the soil, the sun, the rain, the farmer, the factory worker, the retail staff, all of which contribute to our ability to wear a shirt. We can hold an awareness of labor and environmental injustices involving our shirt, as well. All of this is *tariki*.

While our discussion of this Precept has focused thus far on the gratitude we feel when we are the *recipient* of goodness, it is important to realize that another way to practice gratitude is to be thankful for what we can *give* to others. How is *giving* to others a gratitude practice? Why is it so natural that when we do kindness for others, we feel so good? Reiki teachings include the view that we are all *already* interconnected, even though we often forget that truth. So when we are of service to *others*, we call in that vast sense of interconnection in which we feel in accord with all beings and at peace; fully expressing the spiritual aspect of ourselves. We invite you to reflect on a recent time that you gave of yourself to another with no expectation of return. You will realize that although you got nothing in return, you feel a joyful harmonious sense, which is the awareness of gratitude.

Contemplation Exercise to Engage with the 3rd Precept ~ *Practice Gratitude*

Ask yourself with curiosity, care and kindness:

When am I most grateful?
What do I express within myself and outwardly when I practice gratitude?
What do I bring into my life when I practice gratitude?
What do I bring into the world when I practice gratitude?

Contemplate Gratitude and Connect Gratitude with the first 2 Precepts:

When I am filled with anger or worry, I can see that I have no space for anything else.

When I address my anger, worry, and fear, I am creating a space to practice gratitude.

I am mindful of fueling feelings of gratitude instead of fueling my anger and worry, even when it is hard.

Gratitude is a great cure for the mind.
– Hawayo Takata

Happiness is not what makes us grateful.
It is gratefulness that makes us happy.
– David Steindl-Rast

Anecdote: *Tommy's mother introduced herself to Kevin's mom on the preschool playground, saying, "Thank you for your son; Kevin completely changed Tommy's school experience this year." Kevin's mother answered, "Oh, thank you for saying that. How so?" Tommy's mom explained, "My son has cerebral palsy, and your son changed Tommy's life because Kevin included Tommy, and used to wait for him to catch up, and included him with the other children, and that allowed Tommy to make other friends. And seeing your son today, it means even more because I thought your son also had physical limitations, but I see today that he is actually the fastest runner in the group."* When gratitude is felt and expressed it deepens, pointing to the value of deliberately conveying one's gratitude to another person.

Anecdote: With the experience of gratitude, it is sometimes difficult to know who is the giver and who is the recipient. *While doing a surgical rotation, a young doctor was caring for Mr. Larkin, a veteran recovering from a bilateral below-the-knee amputation. On*

Monday morning rounds, the young doctor saw the joy in Mr. Larkin's face when he was reading the Sunday newspaper that was retrieved from the trash by housekeeping. The young doctor knew Mr. Larkin had no family, no visitors, and could not yet move around, so seeing a smile on his face while reading the paper moved her to purchase the Sunday paper and deliver it fresh off the presses to Mr. Larkin on Sunday mornings. For the next two months, while the surgical rotation continued, Mr. Larkin offered a huge smile each time the newspaper was delivered into his hands. When the young doctor saw that smile, she smiled back and went on her way. It appeared on the surface to be a simple exchange, but it was far more than that. When the doctor would see Mr. Larkin's face light up from this simple gesture, she was deeply impacted by his gratitude, feeling a sense of interconnection and peace. This anecdote is an illustration of true *tariki* where it is not possible to distinguish between who is benefitting more from the interaction – giver or receiver – both feel appreciative of kindness and goodness.

4th Precept ~ Live Honestly

What does it mean to live honestly? Living honestly means acting in accord with our deepest values; being open and truthful to our own self and living with purpose. When we live honestly, we give ourselves fully to everything we do. We live intentionally; with awareness of our words and actions. What we mean by our "deepest values" are the true principles that resonate with us; the speech and behavior we want to express; and what is considered most important in our lives. When we think of our truest values, we are uncovering what the authentic meaning and purpose of our lives really is. *In Man's Search For Meaning*, Holocaust survivor Viktor Frankl teaches that finding the meaning and purpose of our lives gives us direction, especially when we face a maze of hardships and uncertainty. Let's explore together how this Precept can support us in connecting to, and expressing, our deepest values so we can live *on* purpose, *with* purpose and spiritual meaning in a way that benefits self and others.

Anecdote: *A neurosurgeon would come home in the evening, yet would call to check on his patients in the middle of the night. I said to him, "That's so kind of you to check on your patients when there already are nurses and doctors in the hospital doing night shifts." When asked, "Why do you do wake up and call to check on your patients even when there are nurses and other doctors in the hospital who can provide coverage for them?" he would reply, "I'm doing this for myself, it makes me feel better. I performed the surgery and therefore I may be able to help out if any questions arise."* By fulfilling his obligation as a doctor, he felt whole because he was living honestly, in accord with his truest values – diligence and integrity – and this is one of the ways he brought meaning and purpose into his life.

In the best of all worlds, we can find a way to live in accord with our values. But don't we know that we do not live in the best of all worlds. Sometimes we have to make compromises between our ideal principles and the realities with which we are faced. We often have to tolerate things that are not in accord with our values. So what can this Precept teach us about everyday constraints on living authentically, and doing what we are meant to do? Knowing full well that we live in a less-than-ideal-world in which compromises will be inevitable, let's agree to honor ourselves and others when we do the best that we can to live with dignity, expressing our truest values in ways that enhance purpose and well-being for self and others.

The 4th Precept reminds us that Living Honestly is the very essence of what living intentionally is all about. Living intentionally ushers in well-being, and well-being brings a deep sense of meaning, fulfillment, purpose, and coherence. Well-being is based on qualities that are embodied in the 4th Precept – Live Honestly – and also echo Aristotle's concept of Eudaimonia. Eudaimonia means living a life of flourishing, full of meaning and purpose. Further, when we Live Honestly, in accord with our deepest values, we actualize deep and authentic connection with others. Part of actualizing our purpose is to go beyond the confines of the self to care and contribute to the well-being of others. Even as we recognize that the world is messy, chaotic, imperfect, and not always pleasant, Living Honestly fosters Eudaimonia because living with authenticity, purpose, and intentionality brings well-being and true mutual human flourishing – mind, body, spirit.

Contemplation Exercise to Engage with the 4th Precept ~ *Live Honestly*

Ask yourself with curiosity, care and kindness:

When am I most able to live in accord with my values?
What does it look like for me to live with intentionality? With purpose? With meaning?
What do I express within myself and outwardly when I am able to live in accord with my values and with purpose?

Contemplate:

How can I do the best I can and honor myself when a compromise is called for between living in accord with my values and the realities of the situation that may limit my choices?

5th Precept ~ *Show Compassion to Oneself and All Beings*

The previous Precepts lead us into the 5th Precept because as our anger, worry, and fear soften, the more we can access the gratitude, integrity, and compassion that are naturally present. Compassion is hardwired into us; it is necessary for human connection which, in turn, is essential for our physical, mental, and emotional well-being. As the Dalai Lama writes:

"Love and compassion are necessities, not luxuries. Without them, humanity cannot survive." Compassion is an emotional response we feel when we see suffering and are moved to ease that suffering. Compassion is said to have three elements (Lesser 2019: 138-139):

- feeling empathy toward what the other is feeling and experiencing;
- understanding those feelings and experiences; and
- being motivated to take action on behalf of another's suffering.

The experience of Being compassionate is a state of being in which we embody empathy, tenderness, and understanding. Showing compassion is how we express those qualities of compassion in words and actions toward ourselves and others: honoring self and others and treating self and others with kindness and dignity. Being and showing compassion create a space for us to live in peace with ourselves and others.

This Precept involves being compassionate to ourselves first. Compassion toward oneself is integral to any mind-body healing practice. With self-compassion, we are acknowledging our own areas of pain and suffering, and then we are offering ourselves the understanding and kindness that help us meet distressing emotions and experiences. When we are gentle, kind, and patient with ourselves, we can release the hold our fears and judgmental mind have on us. By engaging with this Precept, the burden of self-criticism begins to dissolve. We experience a softening within the self, and we reach for ease instead of struggle. When we practice kindness and tenderness toward ourselves, we are better able to extend love and compassion toward others, which is the root of altruism and selfless concern for others. We all have experienced this: When we speak to others with words of compassion and act in compassionate ways, we are expressing our genuine care which, by its very nature, nourishes and heals self and others.

In order to explore compassion it can be helpful to explore its opposite. So we pose this question to you: What are we experiencing, and what are we expressing when we are not compassionate? We are experiencing and expressing separateness and indifference. For example, when we pass by an individual who is experiencing homelessness and is in need, and we find ourselves unsympathetic and keep walking, we are experiencing an uncaring part of ourselves that feels unable to extend compassion toward another human being. We are part of a social system in which we are taught to "rate" the value and worthiness of human beings. Some are seen as deserving of our kindness and compassion, and others are simply not seen as worthy of either one. Tragically, we see evidence of cruelty in the form of racism, transphobia, anti-Semitism, and more, every day. This separation from, and devaluation of, others is at the root of callousness and disregard for essential human dignity and beauty. Practicing compassion is the way we mitigate the harmful mindset of separation and indifference, which has brought about extreme cruelty and suffering.

As we will discuss further in Chapter 11 (The Social Suffering: Reiki Practice & Social Justice), it is compassion that moves us to address social injustices even when the injustice may not appear to affect us directly (Galea 2019: 80). Compassion propels us to see beyond the self and recognize the social, economic, and political conditions that create someone's suffering (ibid).

How do we cultivate compassion? We begin by paying attention to our thoughts and feelings. How? Notice when you may feel callous judgment toward another person. At times like this, hardness has got a hold of us. This is the time to reclaim our capacity for openness and softness. With this awareness, we can sever the grip of judgment and disregard of others. Bringing this Precept into our consciousness reminds us to connect with our inner qualities of gentle kindness, tenderness, and compassion, and expand them beyond the self. When we expand these qualities beyond the self, we experience the antidote to fear, separation and judgment. Thich Nhat Hanh teaches that we can all touch the experience of inter-being. Inter-being means feeling yourself as part of the whole web of life; not separate from other beings. This is the ultimate expression of compassionate connection, caring, and concern for others. This all sounds wonderful, but how do we get there? How do we step into this space of non-judgment and compassion? How do we embody a participation consciousness, feeling part of the one web of reciprocity? As introduced in Chapter 4, The Mindful Pause, we can tenderly ask ourselves: "What would my practice of compassion have me say and do today?"

Anecdote: Ellen has been practicing Reiki mind-body skills for many years and is conscious of different forms of suffering around her. *Walking along a congested city street, Ellen looked ahead and noticed a disheveled older woman stopped in her tracks in the middle of the next intersection. The woman was surrounded by her heavy shopping bags that she could no longer carry. Clearly she had walked a ways already with all of these bags, but had lost her stamina right in the middle of the crosswalk. People bustled past her with no recognition of her distress. Ellen saw the woman's angst and rushed ahead, picked up the bags, and helped the woman safely across the street. They walked together, Ellen continuing to carry the bags, and the older woman chatting about her purchases. Ellen asked her how will she be getting home, and was told she would take a cab. It was a very busy day in the city and Ellen wondered how the woman would ever manage with all her bags and get a cab, so Ellen brought the woman and her bags to an optimal location for flagging down a cab. They waited together until a cab stopped, and Ellen assisted the woman into the cab, with instructions that the driver kindly assist the woman into her home.* This is what care and concern for another human being looks like – a simple act.

To truly cultivate this Precept, Show Compassion to all Beings, we can prepare ourselves by making a conscious and deliberate intent to take a solid seat of non-judgmental listening to others. From this seat we can step back from our own agendas; from our own history of tightly-held biases, fears, and past hurts. It is our task, then, to deeply witness, listen, and attend to what another is saying. As we deeply listen, we learn to recognize the other person's reality as they experience it, instead of as how it reflects onto us. We can take the stance of being intrigued by their story instead of leaping in with our own agendas and judgments. There is some useful restraint involved in this process; we develop our capacity to refrain from reverting to our own repetitive narratives, agendas, and constriction. In this space of deep attention to another person, we overcome our habit of silencing, dismissing, excluding, and erasing others. This is how we invite you to practice the Precept, Be compassionate to all Beings.

Anecdote to illustrate the deliberate and intentional cultivation of compassion: *It was no secret that Melinda complained incessantly. In fact, she complained so much that she drove away her friends and coworkers who no longer could tolerate her constant complaining. Sheila drew the short straw among her coworkers, which meant she would be partnering with Melinda in a major work project. Fortunately, Sheila did self-Reiki practice and, prior to her first meeting with Melinda, took just a few minutes to Pause in stillness, anchor her mind and body, and reflect on the 5th Precept. And then, sure enough, Melinda started in with her complaints about how the room was too cold, the chair hurt her back, the coffee tasted rancid, and on and on. Instead of Sheila's usual rolling of her eyes and feelings of utter frustration and impatience, she connected with her genuine empathy and open listening, and said, "Melinda, it must be really lousy to feel that way."*

Once Sheila heard herself say those words, she felt an openness toward Melinda that she hadn't felt before; a capacity to listen without the old judgments and biases toward Melinda. Sheila was able to shift the focus from her own self-absorbed annoyance to the realities of Melinda's experience. Can we be Sheilas? Can we accompany others without judgment and criticism? Can we claim the compassionate qualities within us? Can we be present for others in this way? You will likely find out for yourself that when you practice compassion in this way, you will invite in greater ease and less struggle, enabling all of us to live in peace with self and others.

Contemplation to Engage with the 5th Precept ~ *Show Compassion to All Beings*

It is up to each of us to take on the responsibility for treating self and others with kindness, compassion, and understanding. It is always possible to reach for inner and outer peace and reconciliation. And we need not wait; it is an expression of compassion to be the one to show kindness first.

Ask yourself with curiosity, care and kindness:

When am I most compassionate to myself? to others?
What do I feel within myself and outwardly when I show compassion?
What do I bring into my life when I practice compassion?
What do I bring into the world when I practice compassion?

Contemplate:

When I become aware of and address my judgmental feelings, I am creating a space to practice compassion.
I am mindful of fueling feelings of compassion and inter-being, instead of fueling feelings of fear and separation, even when it is hard.

Compassion... is spacious and very generous.
When a person develops real compassion,
he is uncertain whether he is being generous to himself or someone
else
because compassion is spacious generosity, without direction,
without "for me" and without "for them."
– Chogyam Trungpa Rinpoche

How each of us behaves in daily life is, after all,
the real test of compassion.
– The Dalai Lama

Anecdote of how our daily life is the real litmus test of compassion: *A physician devoted his life to healing and curing illness. Beyond the requirements of his work, he had infinite compassion toward all he treated. Moreover, he never forgot that the engine of the hospital was the housekeeping staff, telephone operators, secretaries, and nurses, without whom the hospital would not run. He deliberately took extra time to greet everyone with genuine care for their well-being. He consistently reminded his medical students and residents to take the time to listen to each patient, so that patients knew they were being heard. His caring extended beyond the hospital workplace to daily life with everyone he encountered. Even after long work days, he nurtured family, extended family, and friends by giving of himself by listening to each person with sincere concern. Each felt the quality of his supportive, calm presence and care, as he created space for them to be heard.* This kind of being and showing of compassion exemplifies Pure Action, which is when we give of ourselves with no expectation of return.

Chapter 9

The Practice: Suggestions for Your Self-Reiki Practice

This chapter offers some practical ways to bring self-Reiki practice into your life, so it can be a sustainable resource for you every day. We view self-Reiki practice as unfolding in two different contexts. (1) Self-Reiki practice you choose to do as a formal, dedicated practice at a designated time and place. (2) Self-Reiki practice you turn to as a tool in the moment. We will share tips on both, as they complement each other. Let's start with the practice context of a regular, dedicated practice.

To experience the cumulative benefits of Reiki practice for healing mind and body, we encourage you to establish a consistent, ongoing formal practice, tailored to your life and schedule. This will take some preparation, structure, and commitment. Having a routine is helpful, including:

- Holding an intent that you are creating a sustainable practice for yourself.
- Setting aside a designated and comfortable space in your home or elsewhere for your self-practice. You will come to associate this space with your practice time.
- Similarly, you may wish to consider playing beautiful music that you will also come to associate with your practice time.
- Carving out, and building in, a time in your day that fits your schedule.
- Setting a timer for 15, or more, minutes.
- In establishing your formal practice time, building in a consistent place and time each day can be helpful. Your consistent time of day may be upon waking or before bed,

if these options suit your schedule. Some people prefer to set aside time when they return from their day in order to make the transition smoother.

- Build in a time that is convenient and realistic for your schedule so you can follow through with your practice.
- By setting aside a consistent time each day, you are showing your care and compassion for yourself.
- You may choose from among the practices introduced in this book – engaging with the Precepts; *hara* breathing; *Joshin Kokyu-ho*; *Gassho* meditation; 3 Diamonds of *Ki* meditation practices; hands-on self-healing, including the "Reiki Relief Remedy."
- Make a commitment to yourself to set aside at least 15 minutes of practice time each day. To start with, choose any of the self-Reiki practices to which you are drawn. Later, you may find that you add more self-Reiki practices, or you alternate the practices. For example, perhaps you will feel comfortable beginning your practice with hands-on self-Reiki while doing *hara* breathing, and over the days, weeks, or months ahead explore *Joshin Kokyu-ho*, *Gassho* meditation, 3 Diamonds of *Ki* meditations, and contemplation of the Precepts.

If you choose to practice with the Reiki Precepts:

- You may wish to contemplate just the one particular Precept you are struggling with the most in your life right now.
- By working with your chosen Precept, you will be able to become more familiar with yourself and experience how working with this Precept can help you clarify what has a hold on you, and what steps you may feel empowered to take to usher in greater ease. Please refer to Chapter 8 on the Reiki Precepts for specific contemplations and

insights.

- Alternatively, you may wish to contemplate just the one particular Precept that resonates with an inner quality you are trying to cultivate at this moment in your life. Please refer to Chapter 8.
- Another option is to journal any thoughts and/or action steps that come up for you as you contemplate one, or more, of the Precepts.

If you choose to engage with all 5 Precepts at once, you may want to engage in inquiry, reflecting on answers to questions such as:

"When am I most angry?" "Who would I be without fueling my anger?"

"When am I most worried?" "Who would I be without fueling my worry?"

"When am I most grateful?" "What do I bring into the world when I practice gratitude?"

"When am I able to live most honestly?" "What do I bring into the world when I live honestly?"

"When am I most compassionate and kind?" "What do I bring into the world when I practice compassion and understanding?"

"How can this Precept help me address my current struggle, or a larger societal struggle?"

"How can this Precept help me situate myself so that I feel my inner strength and carry on?"

Over time, by experiencing the Precepts as a compass for living your life, you will likely find that your emotions become more regulated, and from there, your words and actions become more skillful. In this way we "invite happiness" and well-being into our daily lives, and extend these to others as well.

Developing your sustainable *hara* breathing practice:
Hara breathing is accessible and user-friendly, with no special preparations or paraphernalia.

- If you are most comfortable sitting, please sit while you do your *hara* breathing. Please lie down, stand up, or walk, if more comfortable for you.
- You may wish to bring to your mind the image of the palm tree introduced in Chapter 3 on *hara* breathing, knowing that you can anchor yourself, and settle mind and body, thereby activating the biological response of down-regulating your nervous system.
- *Hara* breathing instructions include allowing a longer out-breath than in-breath. It may take time to become fully comfortable with this breathing pattern, but we know from experience that, over time, the longer expansive out-breath will become more and more natural to you. Instead of working hard, or forcing the longer out-breath, just allowing the lengthened out-breath to happen without force.
- By maintaining your consistent *hara* breathing practice, the body will more easily move into parasympathetic mode when the going gets tough, and any time a calmer, more settled self is needed.
- You may find that you almost-automatically start *hara* breathing when you practice hands-on healing or when you are contemplating the Precepts. We encourage this!

Suggestions for when you choose to practice *Joshin Kokyu-ho* meditation:

- Keep in your mind that your experience will be one of settling the mind, and cultivating focus and clarity, as described in the snow globe analogy from Chapter 5.

- Approach *Joshin Kokyu-ho* as a mindfulness meditation practice; allowing you to observe your thoughts without judgment, so you feel less tossed about by them.
- On the in-breath, focus on bringing a refreshing, *ki*-filled breath down through the body into the *hara*. Each time you inhale, let your thoughts follow the path of the breath settling down into the *hara* space, grounding and settling.
- On the lengthened out-breath, sense your settled, restored self expanding outward.
- Rest your mind on your capacity for spaciousness, knowing you can become less constricted, more open-minded, and can create an expansive space for yourself and others.
- You may sense that you have created room inside for more awareness and more possibilities.

When you do hands-on self-healing, consider these useful ideas:

- You may want to allow 15 minutes or more for your hands-on-healing practice.
- Remember to find the most comfortable position for yourself, whether that be sitting, standing, or lying down.
- Minimize things that may be distracting to you, and mindfully focus your attention inward by practicing *hara* breathing.
- You may choose to follow the hand-placement protocol as described and depicted in Chapter 6, or you may wish to focus on selected hand placements that you feel drawn to at that time.
- You can even spend your entire hands-on-healing practice time with the "Reiki Relief Remedy" hand placement.
- Whichever hand placements you choose during your practice, hold each placement for several minutes or longer, knowing you are nourishing your being on all levels – physical, mental, emotional, and spiritual. Stillness

of the hands on the body is more important than watching the clock to see how many minutes have passed.

- Sense a calming and nourishing connection between the palms of your hands and your body.
- Whichever hand placements you choose during your practice, your nervous system will settle and shift to calm. You will experience stillness and inner ease in the body.

Embodying Courage: A 3 Diamonds of *Ki* Moving Meditation: If you choose to practice with the 3 Diamonds of *Ki* Meditation, please refer to the meditations in Chapter 7, or, for something new, you are invited to try this standing meditation.

Body Like a Mountain: Stand with feet hip-distance apart, with feet planted firmly on the ground, and hands over the *hara* space. Feel your feet connected to the Earth. As you do *hara* breathing, feel your hips, legs, and feet getting steadier with each breath, like the base of a mountain. Feel your connection to Earth *Ki* as your breath travels downward.

Mind Like the Sky: Continue *hara* breathing, and continue feeling your feet connected with the earth. Now reach your hands comfortably and gently upwards allowing a sense of an open and clear mind, like the Sky. When the body is in a posture of vast openness, the mind knows it.

Heart Like the Ocean: Lower your hands to the center of the chest, feeling the integration of body and mind in the Heart. Then, open your arms forward and out to the sides (like hugging a big tree) and feel your heart vast and expansive, like the ocean. Sense your capacity for inter-being with all.

Close this embodied 3 Diamonds of *Ki* practice by bringing the hands back down to the *hara*, pausing solidly in the present moment, experiencing integration of the 3 Diamonds of *Ki* within your being.

As you may recall at the beginning of this chapter, we introduced two contexts in which we can bring self-Reiki practices into our lives: a formal, dedicated practice, as noted above; and an in-the-moment, informal practice. Our practical suggestions for bringing Reiki practice into your life continue now with the focus shifting from Reiki as a formal practice to Reiki as a tool or skill to be practiced "in the moment."

To refer to Reiki practice as a "tool" means we can call upon Reiki mind-body skills such as *hara* breathing, the mindful Pause, hands-on self-healing, engaging with the Precepts, *Joshin Kokyu-ho*, *Gassho* meditation, and 3 Diamonds of *Ki* meditations, in the moment of need and/or to address acute distress. These practices are always with us as a means of physical, mental, and emotional self-healing in times of injury, pain, anxiety, irritability, impatience, and/or other troubling symptoms. When these difficult moments occur, we may tend to forget that we have our own practical Reiki resources with us at all times – our own breath, our own hands, and our own minds. It is especially important to remember that you are able to use your Reiki skills in times of upset and overwhelm.

Reiki practice in-the-moment, however, does not have to be limited to distressing situations. Enjoying stillness is an end in itself. People talk about self-care so frequently that it can lose its meaning, but we suggest that stopping to Pause in any moment can be how we care for ourselves in the moment. When we simply stop, we make space for our minds to clear and our bodies to settle. In that moment we may even notice things that were hidden to us before.

There are countless examples of when and where you may draw on your Reiki mind-body practices as skills in the moment. We hope the following three examples inspire you to utilize Reiki as a tool in the moment for your well-being.

First, many of us find ourselves gripped with fear when we are in medical waiting rooms awaiting test results for ourselves or others. This is an optimal time to bring in hands-on self-healing and *hara* breathing as tools to lessen anxiety in the moment.

Second, many of us are trapped in busy-ness. We can make a conscious decision to Pause and practice *hara* breathing with *Gassho* meditation to free ourselves from the mindset of busy-ness and shift into stillness to restore our well-being in the moment.

Third, Reiki practice can be supportive of restorative sleep. Sleep is one of the pillars of health, so turning attention to our sleep is a gift we can give ourselves. When we don't get enough sleep, we find ourselves irritable, impatient, less mindful, more reactive to situations, and may even jeopardize our health. Reiki practice before bed can settle the mind and relax the body, allowing the mind to shift into stillness, and the body to unwind, so we can more easily fall asleep. Restful sleep and waking refreshed create the optimal physiological and mental-emotional conditions for living well. In fact, one of the most commonly reported benefits of Reiki is improved sleep.

A Self-Reiki Sleep Practice Tip

So how do we go about calming our minds and body leading to restful sleep?

1. *Lying on your back, allow your body to sink down in the bedding.*
2. *Feel your body safely, securely, and comfortably supported by the bed.*
3. *Begin by placing your hands on the lower abdomen, resting them comfortably on either side of the hara space, so your elbows rest comfortably on the bed, with shoulders and neck relaxed. Feel your body settling.*
4. *Bring your focus to your breath. Begin hara breathing, allowing each in-breath to sink down into the hara space (lower*

abdomen).

5. *Allowing the out-breath to lengthen, lasting a little bit longer than the in-breath.*

6. *Continue with slow hara breaths, focusing gently on your breath going in and going out, and on the abdomen as it rises and falls. As you continue hara breathing, allow mind and body to drop down into deep calm, silence and stillness.*

7. *Bring awareness to your hands on the body, sensing the comfort and warmth.*

8. *If you notice the mind tossed about by thoughts that interfere with sleep, tend gently to the thought, then draw your awareness back to the slow hara breaths, to the sensation of the hands on the body, and the gentle rising and falling of the abdomen.*

9. *As you continue hara breathing, and if it is comfortable and comforting for you, link a gentle and nourishing thought to the lengthened out-breath, such as "may I feel safe," or another comforting thought that calms the mind and settles the body.*

10. *If you feel naturally moved to place the hands elsewhere on the body, gently do so at any time during your self-Reiki sleep practice.*

Our last note about building a sustainable self-Reiki practice is deeply important. When we feel shaken, full of anxiety, and the sympathetic nervous system takes over, it is very challenging to settle down and embrace our self-Reiki practice, but that may be when we need it the most. We have experienced this ourselves on and off through the years, giving into the temptation to either stoically muscle through adversity or spiral into frantic overwhelm. Let's see our way clear to pick up our Reiki self-practice even when we are shaken up and distraught.

Chapter 10

The Challenges: Self-Reiki Practice for Specific Life Challenges & Populations

Reiki practice can be a supportive resource for life challenges many of us face. In this chapter, we have selected specific challenges many of us face, or will face, in our lives. Specific challenges we address in this chapter (in alphabetical order) are:

- Adolescents/Young Adults
- Aging
- Burnout/Moral Injury
- Children
- Illness
- Parenting
- Relationships

Adolescents

What are the specific challenges for this population?

The period of adolescence to young adulthood can be a turbulent time, filled with demands and challenges. Questions of identity, self-worth, safety, and purpose in life, all go with the territory of being an adolescent. The adolescent may also be confronted with relentless demands to accomplish and achieve. Peer pressure, bullying and cyber-bullying, along with the pervasive intrusion of technology, can be crushing stressors. The ever-present threat of neighborhood and school violence that plagues adolescents causes serious safety and security concerns that can result in shock and trauma. Both physical and emotional well-being are jeopardized. Of concern, too, is the toxic information-overload happening as a result of electronic and mobile devices. Glaringly absent from the lives of many youth are built-in opportunities to be still, to unplug, to experience peace of mind, ease, and spiritual well-being.

While our adolescents differ from one another, they all share the wish to grow and to find purpose and joy. And what that might look like will vary from teen to teen. In this section we speak to, include, and embrace all adolescents because every young person can benefit from self-Reiki teachings and practice.

How Can Self-Reiki Be Supportive to Adolescents?

How can the adolescent/young adult connect with their own peace of mind amidst ever-constant pressures and demands? Of course, there are no easy answers, but we strongly feel that the silence and stillness Reiki practice brings will allow the brain to rest from its frantic overload and the body to settle so the adolescent can feel comfortable in their own skin.

Here we offer ways in which Reiki mind-body skills can be supportive to adolescents/young adults as a way to coach themselves through tough times, as well as over the long-term. Through self-Reiki practice, the adolescent/young adult can learn to settle a busy mind, regulate troubling emotions, and relax an agitated body. Self-Reiki practice promotes autonomy, allowing one to use one's own inner resources to create composure and courage on a day-to-day basis. Reiki practice empowers the adolescent to manage emotions, handle stress, improve interpersonal relationships, and build resilience. The adolescent/ young adult can have the power to make self-changes, even if they can't control other things in their lives.

While self-Reiki practice is often done on one's own, encouraging independence and autonomy, we strongly advocate group settings for Reiki mind-body skills practice, where adolescents can also feel the support and encouragement of the collective. Group practice amplifies the experience of stillness and connection every time.

Hara **Breathing:** Whether solo, or in a group context, we suggest *hara* breathing as a first step to settling mind and body. Breathing into the *hara* is really about finding the solid seat within oneself; the firm, sustainable foundation from which to navigate the uncertainties of an adolescent's life. By taking simple *hara* breaths throughout the day, or in a dedicated practice, a teen can restore inner solidity and resilience. The advantage of a formal daily practice of *hara* breathing is that it allows teens to consistently practice staying in control of their thoughts and feelings; to mindfully pause before reacting. From this state of mindfulness one can think more clearly and make more skillful choices, and moreover, touch a sense of spaciousness and connection.

Hands-On Self-Healing: With the mind, emotions, and body becoming settled with *hara* breathing, the second practice we recommend is adding the hands-on self "Reiki Relief Remedy." *Hara* breathing and the "Reiki Relief Remedy" can easily be turned to as in-the-moment strategies for self-regulation, as well as part of an ongoing formal solo or group practice for building resilience. The combination of *hara* breathing and "Reiki Relief Remedy" can help the adolescent/young adult feel more self-assured and comfortable in their own skin. *Hara* breathing allows an adolescent to notice that, while focusing on the breath, their thoughts come and go, come and go, and are not permanent. So, the adolescent comes to understand that, even if things are tough right now, things are impermanent. The adolescent can hold hope that things will change, which is critical for well-being (depression, suicide prevention).

Precepts: The "Just for Today" of the Reiki Precepts is a huge disruptor. How? Adolescents today may face relentless future-oriented pressure, or a sense of hopelessness about the future. Therefore "Just for Today" actually disrupts that paradigm. A "Just for Today" mind-state allows the adolescent to experience a necessary, but neglected, part of themselves: the vitality part; the spiritual part; the playful, spontaneous part; the funny, humorous part. Adolescents have to know that not only is it okay to give themselves a break from external demands, it is necessary for the creation of well-being. What adolescent would walk away from a chance to disrupt the status quo? And while they can't avoid societal burdens, they can give themselves the opportunity to balance these with periods of mindful present-momentness, "Just for Today," immersion. Adolescents may consider engaging in an internal monologue, or self-inquiry, to prompt themselves to get anchored in the here and now. This can be as simple as: "Hey, Mia, let your mind rest, take a *hara* breath, and remember that you don't have to get on the runaway train of worry and fear. There is more to you than that." By engaging in this self-talk, adolescents give themselves permission to express parts of themselves that have been inhibited or constricted.

We encourage schools, after-school programs, and organizations that serve teens to encourage teens to practice their mindful Reiki mind-body skills in group settings with friends and peers. The support of the group will energize each participant, offer social connectedness that can alleviate perceived isolation, anxiety, and depression, and amplify the salutogenic effects of Reiki self-practice.

Aging

What are the specific challenges for this population?
On the societal level, the unpleasant reality is that we live in an ageist culture, in which older people are often devalued, and may even be negatively labeled as "unproductive." While it is true that change is always present in life, with aging we may experience an accelerated rate of change with physical pain and illness; loss of family and friends; and a lessening of our previous energy reserves and abilities. What was once accomplished with

ease may become very challenging. Some days we may navigate aging, losses, solitude, and illness with fear, resistance, bitterness and regret, and other days we act with resilience, courage, and composure.

Some days it feels soul-crushing to let go of the identities and roles we had in the past, and what we were able to accomplish with ease; and other days we are able to accept what is happening with us now, and honor the wisdom and experience we have attained. It is difficult to live with physical and emotional discomfort, as this may take up much of our energy, focus, and attention. In fact, we need not pretend to feel great when we don't; it's okay to not feel great. We can acknowledge our difficulties and sadness, but we don't have to fall into a hole and stay there. We may go forward... or sideways, and even backwards on some days, amidst the challenges of aging. With Reiki self-practice, as we settle our minds and bodies, we may touch an openness to acknowledge the areas of distress, while also discovering new roles, identities, relationships, interests, and experiences that foster joy, meaning, and purpose. When we are able to stand on a platform of wisdom and courage, we can move more intentionally through the uncertainties, vulnerabilities, and fears that come with aging.

How exactly can Self-Reiki be supportive?

Let's create a vision of possibilities while aging – even struggling while aging – that Reiki practice can support. There is a Japanese concept, *arugamama*, which means "things just as they are." Reiki practice can help us be with things as they are, even when they're unpleasant, painful, or uncertain (Klagsbrun 2018). In the stillness of our Reiki practice, we have the opportunity to bring our attention to growth, purpose, and spiritual meaning within the context of "things just as they are." Think of it this way, at our given age we have been able to manage everything that has come up thus far. We have accumulated deep wisdom that provides us with the remarkable capacity to navigate through challenging, unpredictable and uncontrollable events. And we can utilize that wisdom to discover new possibilities with the support of self-Reiki practice. We can continue to navigate through challenges as they are, while exploring avenues of growth, purpose, and flourishing. In the stillness of our Reiki practice, we may be open to rethinking our priorities; recalibrating what is of value to us. Instead of feeling trapped by the challenges that come with aging, we may feel it is possible to hold "dual awareness": to be with things as they are, and move toward what is fresh and nourishing to body, mind, and spirit.

A second Japanese concept, *ikigai*, is helpful to reflect on as we age. *Ikigai* means "our reason for being"; "the things that we live for that allow our possibilities to blossom." *Ikigai* is the source of purpose in our lives; the things that make our lives worthwhile. We know we have found our *ikigai* when our endeavors boost our well-being, and bring us more energy than they take away. We construct spiritual meaning and purpose in our lives, *ikigai*, by choosing to make good use of the time and talents we have. A helpful practice here is to gently inquire into ourselves: "What do I want to pay attention to and invest in?" Whatever we choose to invest our attention and energy in will be nourished. At any age, let's choose to engage in that which nourishes and supports our body, mind, and spirit, our *ikigai*.

Practicing with the Reiki Precepts: Engaging with the Reiki Precepts is a concrete way to reconnect with the deepest values and qualities we have gained from our life experience and accumulated wisdom. If we have the capacity for mindfulness and heartfulness, then we have the capacity for well-being. Remember, we don't overcome our uncomfortable feelings by ignoring them. Rather, we experience well-being when we include mindful awareness of all of our feelings. When we engage with the Reiki Precepts as a compass for our lives, we come to realize that the wisdom and spiritual growth we have gained over our lives matches the wisdom within the Precepts.

Hara **breathing:** On a very practical level, we invite you to practice daily *hara* breathing. The emphasis on the lengthened out-breath reminds us to invite in spaciousness, creating space within ourselves to accommodate the ups and downs that inevitably come with aging.

We encourage you to explore and experiment with daily hands-on self-Reiki practice, practicing the Pause, and engaging with the 3 Diamonds of *Ki* meditations for overall well-being, as well as to address specific conditions ranging from physical aches and pains to daily fears and stresses. You may choose to practice self-Reiki on your own, and we also recommend Reiki self-practice in group settings. These Reiki practice groups may be located in the community, such as at senior centers, local libraries, YMCAs, or within senior residential settings. Experiences of anxiety and depression in later life may be alleviated by group Reiki practice. In our work with Reiki mind-body skills workshops, we have consistently found that group practice, when it is possible, can amplify the benefits of Reiki practice. Perhaps most important of all, is the intent that self-Reiki practice, on one's own, or in a group, sparks the vitality and spirit within that has carried you thus far.

Children: Empowering All Children with Self-Reiki Practice Skills

What are the specific challenges for this situation?
Children will inevitably experience meltdowns, temper tantrums, and bad moods when they encounter disappointments and upsets over which they may have little control. When young children feel powerless, they may try to exert their power in ways that are challenging for them and the adults around them.

Although outbursts are inevitable and expected, they can be completely overwhelming for the child. [Of course, the caregiver also is distressed by the outbursts of the youngsters, but this section focuses on the experience of the child.]

Beyond this, research conducted by Kaiser Permanente and the CDC, beginning in 1995, found that childhood adversity and trauma are linked to physical and mental-emotional illness and disease in adulthood. The Adverse Childhood Experiences Study (ACEs Study) discovered that traumatic or highly stressful experiences in childhood have lifelong adverse emotional, behavioral, and physiological impacts (Felitti et al. 1998). ACEs include adverse experiences that were inflicted on the child directly (physical abuse, verbal abuse, sexual abuse, physical neglect, emotional neglect); and adverse experiences to which the child was exposed in the household or in the community (a parent who is an alcoholic or drug-user, a parent who was a victim of intimate partner violence, a family member who is incarcerated, a family member diagnosed with a chronic mental or physical illness, loss of a parent through death/divorce/ abandonment, unemployment, poverty, homelessness, racism, bullying, neighborhood violence, historical trauma).

The ACEs study demonstrated that ongoing exposure to adverse situations, such as domestic abuse or growing up in poverty, causes the body's natural fight-or-flight stress response to stay switched on. Elevated stress hormones change the functioning of the child's brain, weaken the immune system, and alter the way a child's DNA is read and transcribed. When inflammatory stress hormones flood a child's body and brain, they alter the genes that govern stress reactivity, resetting the stress response to "high" for life. This increases the risk of inflammation, which sets the terrain for cancer, heart disease, and autoimmune diseases later in life. Fortunately, it has also been found that the presence of caring and calming adults, as well as the child practicing mind-body skills that elicit the parasympathetic response, can mitigate the adverse effects of early trauma (Burke 2018).

How can Self-Reiki practice support young children?

Self-Reiki practice is accessible to people of all ages, so, of course, children can learn and practice Reiki mind-body skills for self-calming and self-regulation. There is not a single self-Reiki practice described in this book that a child cannot access. Reiki practices help children calm and settle their body and emotions to bring about a shift into the parasympathetic nervous system. Moreover, children, like adults, deserve and need the opportunity for spiritual expression which self-Reiki practice promotes.

You know how children have play time, story time, bath time, mealtime, and bedtime? We encourage caregivers to also build into the child's day their self-Reiki practice time. Self-Reiki practice time need be as little as 5-10 minutes each day. Caregivers and siblings can also join in the practice with the child. Carving out this special time for a meditative, healing practice in the household will serve the child now and in the years to come. Let's see the possibilities.

The "Stomping" Mindful Pause: A child can access a self-break, or Pause, in any moment of overwhelm or stress. One way to create a space for Pausing is for the child to deliberately and mindfully, but gently, plant one foot on the floor, and then the other, followed by a *hara* breath, to feel themselves solidly grounded. No stomping really needed. A child can repeat this action several times, or simply hold their feet in place for several seconds. This practice creates a sustainable space for Pausing, which down-regulates the nervous system. Even when not in distress, the habit of taking a mindful Pause refreshes and reminds the child of their capacity to slow down and create an inner space which is, at the same time, peaceful and revitalizing for body, mind, and spirit.

Hara **Breathing:** Children can learn the skill of *hara* breathing, which involves a longer out-breath than in-breath, by practicing any of the following exercises: (a) gently blowing soap bubbles in slow motion; (b) pretending to very slowly blow out a birthday cake-full of candles; or (c) blow slowly through pursed lips so a pinwheel slowly turns. Of course an exaggerated blowing will not be effective; rather, a very slow out-breath through pursed lips. Blowing bubbles, blowing out candles, and spinning a pinwheel, all require a lengthened out-breath, just like *hara* breathing. You may recall that it is the longer out-breath that signals the brain to down-regulate the nervous system. The more the child practices *hara* breathing, the easier it is for the child to shift out of hyper-arousal. In addition, the more the caregiver can model *hara* breathing, the more the child will be able to incorporate the practice.

Another fun and pleasing way to move into *hara* breathing is for the child to lie down on their back. Then the child places a bean bag toy on their lower belly area (*hara*). As the child slowly breathes in and out, they learn to experience the difference between a shallow chest breath versus a full belly breath by watching and feeling the bean bag toy on the belly gently moving up and down. Depending on the child's age, the child may wish to count the in-breath for 2 counts, and the out-breath for 4 counts. Once a child learns, and is comfortable with, *hara* breathing, they can bring it into their day-to-day routine, providing a reprieve and a reminder of the settled inner space within.

"Reiki Relief Remedy": We encourage the child to utilize the "Reiki Relief Remedy" hand placement (Chapter 6). The child places one hand on the upper chest and the other one on the solar plexus (where the ribs separate) with light pressure, like a self-hug. The child can access the "Reiki Relief Remedy" anytime and anyplace. For children that feel moved to practice hands-on self-Reiki for longer periods of time, the full hand-placement protocol (Chapter 6) is simple to remember because it goes from head to toe. The child begins by restfully placing the hands on the head, and then moves down the body to the feet, lingering in each hand placement 2-3 minutes, or more, feeling a calming connection between the hands and the body. This sense of connection with the body allows the child a restorative practice that nourishes mind, body, and spirit.

Reiki Precepts

"Just For Today": The Reiki Precepts open with the phrase "Just for Today." "Just for Today" is an expression that can help the child realize an important teaching: when things get rough, the child may think things will always be rough; that things will never change. "Just for Today" helps the child understand that how they feel in this moment is not how they may feel even later in the same day.

"Do Not Fuel Anger": For children, the first Precept, "Do Not Fuel Anger," can be used as a self-awareness reminder to sense feelings of anger as they bubble-up, acknowledging that anger is a natural emotion to experience. Not only that, the Precepts help children realize that feelings of anger are just one part of them, there is so much more, and they do not have to fuel their feelings of anger. When children practice self-awareness of their emotions (such as anger), and self-control of their actions, they will certainly feel better about themselves, and grow in wisdom about their feelings and how they relate to others.

"Do Not Fuel Worry": It is natural for children to experience fear, worry, and uneasiness. While worry can drain adults, it can take the childhood right out of the child. This Precept can help a child understand that, although they cannot control external circumstances, they can influence their own inner state by acknowledging, but not fueling their worry. A helpful way to not fuel worry is to practice *hara* breathing, which will shift the nervous system to a more restful state, and create a peaceful inner space. When the child becomes more settled, they can recognize that fear and worry are normal and natural parts of life. Knowing that it is okay to have worry will defuse the tension that the child experiences and will soften the impact of the worry, and even allow the child to feel comfortable sharing their fears and worries with grownups in their lives.

"Practice Gratitude": This Precept serves as a reminder to the child that, even when life feels overwhelming, they can slow down and actually take stock. Cultivating appreciation requires that we first take notice. Caregivers can help children notice possibilities for experiencing appreciation. By modeling expressing awe at people and things they find meaningful, caregivers can be living examples of "Practicing Gratitude." If this kind of noticing is sustained by the caregiver, a child will mirror the practice. In this way, the child can connect with their own developing sense of spacious appreciation for the people and things around them.

"Live Honestly": The fourth Precept encourages the child not to be swayed by the crowd, and by values that are not truly their own. Rather, to look within, take stock, and be honest with themselves to find and experience their own purpose and direction. It is extremely difficult for children to not cling to approval and validation, so we encourage adults to model loving acceptance and support of children who follow their own path, are true to their own way, even if it is not the norm.

"Show Compassion to Oneself and All Beings" supports the child in prioritizing self-compassion in the face of over-the-top societal expectations, as children can be very hard on themselves. Further, when children take on the responsibility of treating others with kindness, compassion, and understanding, they feel better about themselves, more spacious and connected.

It may be fun and helpful for the caregiver to give the younger child the Precepts printed on a piece of paper, which the child can decorate. A valuable exercise is for the younger child to consider each Precept and how it can apply to real-life situations in their life or in other people's lives. It may be useful for the child to choose one Precept a day or one Precept a week for this exercise. Talking about, and applying, the Precepts with the child can be a way the child learns life lessons that they can incorporate into their daily lives.

The 3 Diamonds of *Ki*: Although the 3 Diamonds of *Ki* meditation may seem like it is for adults, it is actually very child-friendly! For "Body Like a Mountain," a child can visualize and proclaim themselves being as solid and strong as a mountain. Children can sense what it feels like to be as stable and steady as a mountain. They may even want to draw a mountain, create a story, pretend they are a mountain, or do physical movements that convey the feeling of being sturdy and grounded. For "Mind Like the Sky," a child can visualize and proclaim their heads feel clear, vast, and free like the sky. Again, they may wish to draw a sky, create a story, pretend they are like the sky, or do physical movements that convey the feeling of being open, spacious, and at ease. For "Heart Like the Ocean," a child can visualize and proclaim their heart feels as connected to others as the waves in the ocean. They may even want to draw an ocean, create a story, pretend they are an ocean, or do physical movements that convey the feeling of being connected to others, animals, and nature. We recommend that the child specifically names the people and beings to whom they feel connected, as this encourages awareness and noticing of connection.

Anecdote of the proverbial supermarket scene: There are times when unexpected and challenging behavior arises. *Imagine a child being in a busy, crowded, overwhelming supermarket. The child has had enough and wants to leave. The checkout line is quite long and, of course, the child doesn't really understand they have to wait in line and pay before they leave. The child starts to scream "go home." The caregiver tries to explain that they must pay for the groceries first. However, all the child is experiencing is the overwhelming noise and crowd, and their sympathetic nervous system is spiraling out of control. The caregiver Pauses, recognizes and honors the child's legitimate feelings – the child is overheated in their jacket; overstimulated by the loud, annoying music that customers must shout over to be heard; and overloaded by the bright, glaring lights. The caregiver remembers to suggest to the child to pretend they are smelling the roses, and then blowing out a lot of candles on a birthday cake with a long, slow out-breath to make sure they get all the candles out. As the child "smells the roses" and "blows out the candles" a few times, along with the caregiver's modeling, their body shifts into parasympathetic mode. The caregiver then suggests that the child give themselves a hug with the "Reiki Relief Remedy." By the time they are ready to check out, the child is calmer, and even playful, and the caregiver is able to pay for the groceries.*

This is one example in which a caregiver was faced with an overwhelmed child. The Reiki practices the caregiver modeled, and that the child was able to do, are surprisingly simple, yet can be immensely helpful for both of them in de-escalating the child's overwhelm. One may think that once a child goes into "overwhelm mode," it is too late to do anything but endure it or abandon the groceries and exit. Although each child has different ways of settling, the "Reiki Relief Remedy" and *hara* breathing in the moment are definitely worth a try. Further, when these skills have been practiced at home, the child is more readily able to move into a settled inner space at other times.

Personal health is related to self-control;
self-control brings with it happiness.
Maria Montessori

Illness

Illness sets up a cascade of hardship and pain. Illness can range from a slight cold to being critically ill, all of which can involve suffering. Along with illness comes overwhelming anxiety, fear, constriction, and feelings of vulnerability. Anxiety grips us with concerning questions: How long will this illness last? What if I don't get better? Will I ever get "back to myself"? Furthermore, fears dominate our thoughts in an immense cascade: fear of not being able to continue with our daily routine; fear that our illness will prevent us from working; fear of financial instability; fear of pain; fear of not being able to take care of our children or elderly parents; fear of not being able to take care of ourselves and becoming dependent; fear of being isolated; fear that others will treat us differently; fear of death. Illness has a domino effect on all aspects of our lives, and also on the lives of our loved ones.

When we are ill, our physical and cognitive abilities may be impaired, preventing us from accomplishing the routine tasks and activities of daily life. Our entire lives can be affected in one abrupt moment. The disruption and disability illness causes range from minor inconveniences to our lives potentially being turned upside down. How do we deal with illness and the harsh realities that go along with it?

How can Self-Reiki practice support us through illness?

What can help us get through even the most difficult of times? Facing an illness brings deep suffering and yet calls on us to reclaim our inner courage and strength so that we can go forward with our treatment and, if possible, recovery. When we are ill we live in the midst of fearful uncertainty, yet we can practice self-Reiki to support us so that we can manage the uncertainty and disturbing thoughts and feelings with strength of mind. Self-Reiki practices strengthen our ability to develop an inner stability, even when facing the complexities of illness and of how we feel about our illness. Reiki mind-body skills give us "the strength to be" (Dietrich Bonhoeffer); to refocus and reclaim our lives; to help us get through some of the most difficult of times as we embody our courage from within. And, of course, during those times when we are ill and feel as though we are falling apart, our Reiki mind-body skills can help us regain our footing; enhancing awareness that any impairments we are currently experiencing exist side-by-side with sources of resilience and spiritual strengths we possess.

In addition to helping us connect to inner strength, self-Reiki practices also positively impact our physiology. By facilitating a shift from the sympathetic to parasympathetic nervous system, self-Reiki practices can reduce the levels of stress hormones in the body; lessen inflammatory processes; improve immune function; and reduce the perception of pain. Moreover, what happens physiologically is deeply interconnected with our psychological processes. Reiki mind-body practices help us cultivate resilience and adaptive responses to the cascade of psychological distress. When we are in the grip of mental-emotional pain, our world can become very small. The poet and philosopher, Mark Nepo, points to the experience of spaciousness that may be available to us: "When in pain, try to enlarge your sense of things." When considering Mark Nepo's teaching, we can see why pet therapy is effective; why a visit from caring people helps us feel better; and why hospitals employ chaplains of all faiths. All of these enlarge our perspective at the very moment when our world can shrink.

When faced with illness, we suggest any combination of these 4 comforting self-Reiki practices:

Hara **breathing practice:** When we are ill, *hara* breathing can help us get through tough moments by anchoring our bodies, soothing our emotions, and enlarging our sense of things. *Hara* breathing activates the parasympathetic nervous system, thereby promoting calm and healing.

Hands-on Healing: We also encourage you to turn to hands-on self-Reiki every day. Hands placed on the affected areas of one's body, or elsewhere on the body where we feel drawn to place our hands, may address pain and discomfort, as we tend to our needs in a comforting and caring way.

Precepts: Engaging with the Precepts may be helpful as well. We invite you to choose the Precept that feels right for you in any moment during your illness and recovery. A helpful practice here is to gently inquire within ourselves: "What do I want to pay attention to at this very moment?" "How can this Precept help me situate myself so that I feel and claim my inner strength to carry on?"

Gassho **meditation** makes no demands of us, as it brings us into a nourishing stillness.

Please keep in mind that Reiki is a healing practice, as opposed to a curing practice. To cure means to eliminate all evidence of disease; to heal means to become whole. Even if one is not cured, one can still feel whole with Reiki practice. The experience of healing is when one's sense of self remains intact and whole despite any mind-body limitations, discomfort, and uncertainties that come with illness. If we are living with a chronic condition that cannot be cured, such as osteoarthritis, Reiki practice can bring healing by reducing the grip that feelings of helplessness and fear have on us. It is possible to feel a sense of wholeness even when the rug has been pulled out from under us. We gain a perspective that just because one thing is broken doesn't mean everything is broken (Doty 2017). We can put our attention on the parts of us that feel good enough, including our spiritual self, helping us to feel whole despite our illness. It's about where we place our attention.

For example, we can bring our hands and our awareness to parts of the body that feel neutral or easeful and be mindful of the fact that there is give and take and balance between places of discomfort and places of ease. That is the experience of healing. Medical treatments are a necessity when we are ill, of course, yet there are some aspects of the illness experience that medical science cannot address. Reiki practice encourages a shift from pain to possibility. What possibility? The possibility of finding courage and spaciousness in the midst of distress, challenges, and uncertainty; the possibility of recognizing our capacity to act in affirming ways; the possibility of cultivating the sacred within the everyday.

Anecdote: *Mark, an otherwise healthy, fit, young bank teller, went on a mountain-bike adventure weekend. After the 3-hour car ride home, his back muscles were in such a tight spasm that he could not straighten up. Stooping over in intense pain, Mark got himself into his apartment. All he could do was lie down flat on the floor. Fortunately, his phone was still in his pocket and he was able to call his friend and neighbor, Roger. Roger came over and got Mark some ice and ibuprofen, and offered any further assistance Mark needed. Mark felt that all that could be done was being done. When Roger left, it suddenly dawned on Mark that he could practice the Reiki mind-body skills he had learned at a Reiki self-practice workshop to ease his distress. As Mark settled into hara breathing with his hands resting on his torso, he felt himself drop down beneath the fear of, and resistance to, the pain. In physiological terms,*

Mark was experiencing a down-regulation of his nervous system. Self-Reiki practice got Mark through the acute injury phase, along with rest, ice, and ibuprofen, after which Mark chose to commit to physical therapy. His healing was slow going. What kept Mark feeling whole despite the debilitating, recurrent back problem, and the slow process of recovery, was the support he experienced from his self-Reiki practice. Mark had learned that self-Reiki practice brings cumulative benefits, so he developed a consistent go-to self-practice routine, along with his Physical Therapy Home Exercise Program. His self-Reiki practice allowed Mark to tap into patience he never knew he had, and persevere through the arduous healing process with courage, composure, and resilience. Throughout this process, although Mark was not cured, as he still at times experienced pain and physical limitations, his sense of self was intact and whole. That is what healing feels like.

Workplace Burnout and Moral Injury

What are the specific challenges for this situation?

In 2019, the World Health Organization's International Classification of Diseases (ICD-11) included burnout as a medical diagnosis. Burnout is included in the ICD-11's section on employment/unemployment-related problems. Given that workplace burnout is now a legitimate medical diagnosis, doctors can diagnose someone with burnout if they experience: (1) feelings of energy depletion or exhaustion, (2) increased mental disturbance from their job or feelings of negativism or cynicism related to their job, (3) reduced professional efficacy, despite a high level of responsibility.

Health care providers, first responders, emergency workers, firefighters, teachers, and others experience high rates of burnout due to excessive workloads and time pressure; high levels of responsibility; reduced autonomy; high-demands combined with low control; morally distressing situations;

and sense of professional ineffectiveness. People experiencing workplace burnout may feel physical and emotional exhaustion, loss of meaning and purpose in their work, anxiety, depression, and an overall sense of hopelessness. Workplace burnout takes a toll on our reserves of strength and well-being. Burnout is "an erosion of the soul" (Maslach 2003, cited in Epstein 2017: 160). While the CDC has limited the medical diagnosis of burnout to the workplace, it is critical to note that burnout as an "erosion of the soul" can be more pervasive. Burnout is not limited to the workplace, but rather can affect people who are unemployed, students, parents, patients, carers, immigrants, and stigmatized groups.

Before we discuss strategies for well-being with Reiki practice, it is imperative to highlight that burnout is an individual-level experience within what is a pervasive systemic, organizational problem in our workplaces and in society at large (Langade et al. 2016). Given this lens on the burnout experience, researchers refer to the concept of Moral Injury, first applied in relation to returning Iraq and Afghanistan combat veterans. Moral Injury occurs when one's moral compass, beliefs, conscience, and values are damaged by harmful workplace policies, demands, and constraints. Morally injured employees, further, feel unable to perform their duties and attend effectively to those they serve. While recognizing this critical reality, we know that advocating for and bringing about systemic, organizational change will take time. In the meantime, engaging with self-Reiki practices to restore purpose, meaning, value, and connection can begin right now. And, further, may motivate us to be advocates and activists for more upstream system-wide changes.

How exactly can Self-Reiki practice be supportive?

Self-Reiki practice can assist us in cultivating strengths in the face of intense emotions that workplace burnout and moral injury may bring. Our practice can nurture self-awareness of our thoughts, emotions, and reactions. Beyond this, we nourish the capacity to hold intentional presence, bringing our professional knowledge and skills, as well as compassionate care, to those we serve.

An important component of burnout and moral injury is neglecting to care for oneself which has consequences for our overall well-being, as well as for those we assist (Sapiro 2018). While stress wears down all the systems of the body, burnout crushes the soul (Sapiro 2018). Reiki practice can nourish and replenish mind, body, emotions; literally restoring inner resources and reserves. The self-regulation and resilience that Reiki practice can bring is a supportive source of strength when we feel burned-out and harmed by the systems in which we work. Moreover, when one is in a settled state, one is better able to notice the emerging signs and symptoms of burnout within oneself. It is imperative that Reiki practice be utilized as an early self-care intervention in the burnout process in order to prevent burnout from developing into depression, poor coping, chronic stress, hopeless and helpless feelings, and physical illness.

Reiki practice is an antidote to the many dimensions of burnout. In the physical dimension, while burnout brings sympathetic nervous system activation, inflammation, and impaired immune function, Reiki practice facilitates parasympathetic nervous system activation, reduced inflammation, enhanced immune function, and the optimal functioning of the systems of the body. In the mental-emotional dimension, with sustained Reiki practice, we can reclaim and build strengths that burnout and demoralization can take away. When we connect with a stable sense of our own health and well-being, we contribute to alleviating the suffering of those we serve and our coworkers, as well as the ability to improve the larger organizational culture.

We invite you to explore and experiment with both in-the-moment self-Reiki practice while at work, as well as formal daily self-Reiki practice at home. We especially encourage you to consider practicing *Gassho* meditation in conjunction with *hara* breathing. In this combined practice, raise your hands into *Gassho* position, at heart level, with your fingertips just under the nose. Bring your focus to the sensation of the lengthened out-breath from your nostrils as it passes over the point where the middle fingers meet. Allow any other thoughts and sensations of mind and body to shift/move into the background. As you continue with the one-pointed focused concentration *Gassho* meditation, you will be able to reclaim your own direct experience of stillness and steadiness, despite the harm workplaces can bring. When thoughts of "what-ifs" draw you in, you don't have to get lost in them; instead choose to gently persevere in returning your attention to the sensation of the lengthened out-breath passing over the middle fingers.

For those of us feeling the distress of workplace burnout, the Precepts offer a harbor in the storm. Sitting in mindful contemplation of the Precepts, feelings of anger, worry, fear, and impatience are more easily recognized. Further, we may gain understanding into what gives rise to these feelings about our workplaces, our coworkers, patients, students, customers. When we acknowledge and accept these mind-states of anger, worry and fear, we come to know that we do not have to fuel them. We may experience more ease instead of struggle, strengthening our resolve to address moral injury for ourselves, and for the sake of our coworkers and those we serve.

Parenting

What are the specific challenges for this population?
The responsibility of raising a child to become an independent, emotionally resilient adult can be formidable. All parents experience concerns about their children's development and well-being, and can benefit from Reiki teachings and practices. On the one hand, experiencing children's smiles, laughter,

and joyous moments can fill the parent's soul with happiness beyond description and a sense of deep fulfillment. When the child/adolescent is doing well, the parent has a sense of ease. On the other hand, when the child/adolescent is struggling, the parent can experience alarm, dread, and fear. Alarm, dread, and fear are strong emotions that we intensely feel in our bodies. Both child and parent suffer: The child/adolescent perceives the parent's stress, inevitably amplifying emotional distress, creating a vicious cycle for both.

As parents, our task is to hold a secure space for the child to grow, without burdening them with our worries. This task is not easy, as a parent must be able to handle their own anxiety while being well aware that the child/adolescent may be struggling. When parents can hold the necessary calm space, the child/adolescent is able to model the parent's behavior and grow with resiliency toward independence. Imagine this: You are the parent of a child who is struggling and not meeting the normative developmental and academic milestones. Your natural emotional reaction is worry and fear about the child's well-being, security and future. Worry and fear, although understandable, drain you and, moreover, are not what your child needs from you. Instead of getting caught up in emotional turmoil, parents can turn to Reiki practice to lessen the grip of worry and fear. In this way, parents become more available to their children and also better equipped to approach any challenges with a clear heart-mind. With self-Reiki practice, parents can become the model of a steady platform of courage for the child/adolescent, thus increasing resilience for both parent and child. [Of course, there is so much more to the parenting experience than struggle, but here we are addressing the challenges.]

How exactly can Self-Reiki practice be supportive to the parent/caregiver?

Parents can learn and benefit from Reiki mind-body skills to address and navigate their strong emotions. These Reiki strategies can be an antidote to a parent's worries and fears, helping us calm and steady so we can weather the storms that come with all stages of parenting. When our mind-body settles, we can think clearly and parent more skillfully. We have all been in situations where the appropriate thing for us to do is to advocate for our child/adolescent's needs. It is optimal to advocate from a steady mind-body state. Reiki self-practice allows us to feel settled within, so if and when our parental advocacy is called upon, we will have a more purposeful effect. Best practice is for parents reading this book to review the chapters on the Reiki practices (*hara* breathing, the Pause, *Joshin Kokyu-ho*, *Gassho* meditation, hands-on self-Reiki, the Precepts, the 3 Diamonds of *Ki*) and explore the best fit for you.

By now it is clear to our parent-readers that by Pausing and taking slow, deep *hara* breaths we can down-regulate our nervous system, thereby settling our emotions, thinking more clearly, and bringing supportive calm to ourselves. Similarly, hands-on self-healing for 10-15 minutes, or 3 Diamonds of *Ki* practice, can help manage the cascade of overwhelming emotions and access our inner composure and balance. Parental worry and fear can take up so much emotional space that it is difficult for a parent to claim the strengths that lie within them. Reiki self-practice allows the parent to access the wisdom and understanding that may have been covered up by overwhelm, worry and fear.

An amazing benefit of our self-Reiki practice as parents is that as we calm and find our strengths, so too the child calms... and it works! The parent's own emotional resilience "serves as a template for a child to see how to deal with challenges, and how to understand their own emotions" (Siegel 2018). In fact, the child synchronizes their own heart rate and breathing with the parent's, allowing the child to also pause and take stock of their own emotions (Lewis 2018). Children learn, and benefit from, these skills best when their parents/caregivers model them. We encourage "dual generation" mind-body interventions, where parents, teachers, coaches, and other caregivers, together with the children, learn self-regulation skills, creating collective growth and resilience.

One of the difficult tasks of parenting is to give the child enough space to flourish despite our worries and concerns. When parents practice self-Reiki, they may feel better equipped to discern when to step in and when to give the child/adolescent space. We struggle to give our children the necessary space because we tend to fear the worst. When we are in that fearful state of mind, we may forget to Pause and put on the brakes; feeling propelled to step in, fix everything, and rescue the child. One of the most significant benefits of Pausing and *hara* breathing for parents is putting a brake on our impulse to fix and control, especially when these may not be needed or warranted. When we Pause, we give our children the space to express themselves without us jumping in. We give ourselves and our children the gift of listening deeply to what they are experiencing.

Relationships: Managing Difficult Relationships
(Note: this section does not refer to situations of interpersonal or intimate-partner violence, for which professional medical and/ or legal intervention may be necessary.)

What are the specific challenges we face navigating difficult relationships?
We often encounter people in our lives that challenge, provoke, and disturb the core of our being. How do we manage to stay settled when others "push our buttons"? Can we disengage from turmoil when we are confronted with people in our lives that provoke hurt? How do we prevent other people's criticism and negativity from affecting our own peace of mind? It is easy to feel angry, disappointed, confused, and hurt by complicated relationships. When we encounter unprovoked and unexpected

behaviors from others, it can feel like an emotional ambush that can push us off balance. How do we avoid getting burned by the intense feelings that are evoked by difficult interactions with others? This section focuses on maintaining our own wholeness and spaciousness in the face of difficult relationships.

How exactly can Self-Reiki practice be supportive in difficult relationships?

We all have experienced unkind behavior from another person. On one end of the spectrum is the example of a stranger unexpectedly speeding by our car to pass us, leaving us with a feeling of shock and vulnerability. We can recover from this type of incident rather quickly as we do not take it personally. This reckless driver probably does this all day long to many people. In other words it is not personal. Some soft *hara* breathing may be all we need to get us quickly back on track feeling steady in our mind/body. However, on the other end of the spectrum, what if it does feel personal? It is not so easy to calm and steady our mind/body when we feel personally attacked by someone with whom we have an ongoing relationship. For our own health and well-being, we have to be mindful of *our own* reactions, and mindful of how *we* are going to relate to our own experience. Reiki self-practice can help us in two ways: First, becoming mindful of *our own* emotions with caring self-awareness; and second, reclaiming emotional wholeness and balance despite caustic interactions with others.

Self-Reiki practice offers us valuable tools for navigating difficult relationships; preventing entanglement in the drama that some individuals may bring into our lives. The more we practice self-Reiki, the more mindful we become of *our* thoughts, feelings, motivations, and expectations. We also become more conscious of our reactions to *other* people's words and actions. Our practice anchors us so we are not tossed about by other people's hurtful behavior. Ultimately mindful Reiki practice helps us learn to *not suffer* from others' provocations.

The first thing we suggest for managing strong emotions when confronted with challenging personalities is to step back, Pause, and practice *hara* breathing. Putting on the emotional brakes with the Mindful Pause, and calming our minds with *hara* breathing, prepares us for an encounter with a difficult individual. The Pause and *hara* breathing allow us to cultivate an inner terrain of emotional balance, thereby preventing the harmful effects of the "fight or flight" response. Imagine going into a meeting with a difficult coworker; why not engage the Pause and start your *hara* breathing *prior* to the meeting. *Hara* breathing gives us the inner calm to acknowledge our strong intense feelings, as well as the clarity to know that we need not fuel them. In this way we can more deliberately *choose* how to respond in ways we may not have considered prior to our Reiki practice. When we set aside time to feel settled and whole by Pausing, putting on the brakes, and *hara* breathing, we are giving ourselves an opportunity to choose ways to distance ourselves from the chaos, while keeping a valued relationship intact.

Anecdote: *Jason was very excited about his engagement to Erica and was eager to announce his plans to his parents. Jason and Erica had been living together in a different city from Jason's parents for almost a year and his parents were always pleased to see Erica when they visited. This always reassured Jason because his parents were typically critical of him and his choices. When Jason conveyed his good news, instead of being joyful for his happiness, Jason's parents started in with their criticism of Erica. Jason felt disappointed and hurt because his parents had been accepting of the relationship up to now. He felt emotionally ambushed and unsettled. In order to settle himself and relate intentionally and consciously to the interaction, Jason took advantage of his Reiki self-practice skills. A few moments of hara breathing and pausing in stillness allowed Jason to gain some emotional balance. This more settled mind-state provided Jason with* *the capacity to think with clarity and discernment about options and choices for responding to his parents.* This anecdote teaches us that ongoing self-Reiki practice helps us become ever more mindful and self-aware of our thoughts and emotions, so we can respond effectively when faced with conflict.

Since our lives will be punctuated by difficult interactions, setting aside time to contemplate the Reiki Precepts can help us gain insight into our own emotional state so we can speak and act skillfully when distressing interactions arise. For example, contemplating the first Precept, Just for Today Do Not Fuel Anger, allows us to put our minds to work *for* us and gain insight into our anger. We may notice that anger arises when we grasp onto what cannot be in a relationship; when our desires and expectations in an interaction are not met. In difficult relationships, in which we have endured the hurtful behavior of others, we may feel entitled to, and justified in, our anger. But justifiable anger is still anger. And fueling anger can still be poison and constrict our mind, body, and spirit, as well as mask distress that may lie beneath the anger (such as feelings of deep sadness, hurt, and disappointment). Let's face it, as hard as it is to tolerate an angry person, try to remember that *we* don't have to live in anger with an angry person.

Chapter 11

The Social Suffering: Reiki Practice & Social Justice

While we strongly encourage committing to daily self-Reiki practice for our *own* sustenance, the practice also encourages and supports us in the work of repairing the world so that *all* people can feel nourished and thrive. When we work with our own minds and bodies, with our own conditionings and biases, we naturally expand from self-concern to concern for others. We are strengthened to touch our own biases and conditionings around issues of systemic inequality, structural racism, gender bias, and classism, among others (Rhonda Magee 2018). Although we face the challenge of living in a society that is structured to push us apart; a society that continues to struggle with racism, sexism, and all the other isms (Rhonda Magee 2018), we cannot acquiesce to the abuse of human rights.

Looking inward all by itself cannot be the sole solution to social, economic, and political forces beyond the control of individuals. Unfortunately, it is *not* true that every individual has the power to be what they want to be and make happen what they want to happen. Instead, larger structural forces, policies, and institutions limit and constrain an individual's capacity to exercise resilience and reach for wellness. Resilience and resilience-building do not occur in a vacuum. We need to ask what is happening "out there"; what are the historical and social conditions that are consistently challenging resilience and coping skills, especially of those most structurally disempowered. Social epidemiologists, Wilkinson and Pickett (2011), have demonstrated that socioeconomic inequality, including that caused by racism, is consistently correlated with poor physical and mental health and wellness; and the greater the degree of inequality in a society, the greater the suffering, harm, and despair.

While Reiki self-practice in and of itself will not address the larger structural forces, such as inequality, that bring harm and disadvantage, there is encouraging news. The Reiki self-practices described in this book support a state of mindful and heartful compassion and courage propelling us to go out there and take action to overcome social suffering, as we transcend the confines of the conditioned self. The suffering of others may no longer be a headline that we merely glance at before moving on to the next item in the news cycle or self-focused project. With a participation consciousness, we move beyond self-growth to collective growth embedded in compassion. If we want love and peace, we have to create it in the world around us (Doty 2017). We have to embody the wisdom and teachings that come from experience:

As you press for justice, be sure to move with dignity and discipline, using only the instruments of love.
– Dr. Martin Luther King, Jr.

Justice is what Love looks like in public.
– Dr. Cornel West

When "I" is replaced by "We," even Illness becomes Wellness.
– Malcolm X

While larger US cultural norms and social structures tend to reinforce individualism and separation, our Reiki practice can usher in a more inclusive sense of engaging with the world. The wounds of *all* people are felt as our own when we open our hearts to the experience of all humanity. The raw wounds felt by so many touch our natural capacity for compassion. Reiki self-practice supports and strengthens us to take our place in what may be difficult conversations about race, class, gender, and social injustice, instead of fearing and avoiding them. We can aim high, too, in terms of taking a stand to oppose the harmful effects of social injustice, racism, and inequality and take on anti-oppression and anti-racism work. When we bring together mindful stillness (*misogi*/the inner) and compassionate action (expansion/the outer), we can contribute to dismantling the ways of thinking and organizing society that have resulted in oppression, causing deep suffering and pain (Rhonda Magee 2018).

We are saying here that we can experience Reiki practice as more than a personal system of teachings and practices. Rather, our commitment to daily consistent practice brings the capacity to be present with all things with honest awareness, including the social structures that separate, exclude, erase, silence, disempower, and bring suffering, in order to build a more just world. As we become more consciously aware with Reiki self-practice, we can recognize the structures and institutions in society that create and sustain harm, and aspire to fulfill our responsibility for collective well-being (Galea 2019: 81). Each of us, in our own way, and together, can be an outward-facing, public face, of what is possible with Reiki practice. With self-Reiki practice we expand beyond the self to see the world with new eyes. When we are free from self-absorption and self-importance, we are open to caring for all others, for choosing to work for an equitable, just, and sustainable world.

Self-growth, development and meditation are just the beginning; these must be balanced by active social engagement and compassionate actions.
– Lama Surya Das

Chapter 12

Conclusion – The Platform For Peace: Sustaining Well-being with Self-Reiki Practice

Reiki practice is not only about addressing pain and suffering, but it is about the creation of well-being and ease. With self-Reiki practice, we develop inner resources and qualities that sustain and nourish our well-being – mind, body, spirit. What does well-being feel like? Well-being feels like being at ease with oneself and calling on our inner resources of mindfulness, resilience, purpose, vitality, and spiritual strength. When we claim these inner resources, we find the courage to be intentionally present with what life brings to us and what we bring to life. Further, *our* courage has a ripple effect on: (a) the well-being of those *around us* by providing *them* with *our* anchored presence, and allowing *them* to find *theirs*; and (b) as Chapter 11 introduced, on our capacity to engage in advocacy and compassionate action to restore justice and bring an end to social suffering.

Mikao Usui, who developed the system of Reiki, wrote: *"The intent of our lives is to achieve a peaceful and joyful mind-body state and then, while holding that peace within, fulfill our purpose."* So we see there is an inner state of well-being to be cultivated (*"a peaceful and joyful mind-body state"*) and from that inner state of well-being, we are open and available, and expand outward through our actions in the world. Sounds great, right? But with lives full of uncertainty and hardships, how do we really cultivate a calm mind and settled body, and move into this *peaceful and joyful mind-body state* that Usui refers to? How do we stay present and available, build courage and composure, in the midst of uncertainty?

Let's take a brief look back and highlight the Reiki practices introduced in this book and see how we can engage with them to sustain ease, well-being, and spiritual expression in addition to addressing pain and suffering on multiple levels.

The Reiki Precepts (Ch. 8): The 5 Reiki Precepts are a compass, pointing the way to cultivating mindfulness and a peaceful way through the world. As discussed in Chapter 8, the first 2 Reiki Precepts (Do Not Fuel Anger and Do Not Fuel Worry) speak to the anger, worry, and fear that can constrict us, keeping us distant from others. Nonetheless, we cannot and should not really escape or avoid these constricting emotions (Reiki self-practice is not about "blissing out"). To the contrary, the Precepts help us *sit with*, and figure out how to *relate to*, our anger, worry, and fear. With this mindfulness, we gradually untangle the knots of anger and worry in our minds, like untangling and freeing a knotted necklace chain until it falls free and takes its natural shape. Practicing the last three Precepts (Gratitude, Honesty, Compassion) invites us to open to what is possible, steering us in the direction of inter-being, spiritual connection, and a sacred participation with all beings with the intent of reducing pain, suffering, and injustice. It is in our everyday life that we really put the Precepts into practice. Meditating on the Precepts is like our lab work; everyday life is our fieldwork, where we apply the Precepts with our words and actions. The more we practice embodying the Precepts, the more natural it becomes to speak and act in ways that honor self and others day-to-day.

When we practice with the Precepts, we reclaim the peace, happiness, and lightness we already have.
– Thich Nhat Hanh

Hara **Breathing** (Ch. 3): *Hara* Breathing is the foundational meditative breathing practice in the system of Reiki. Chapter 3 offered a visual of a palm tree in a storm, whose base is rooted and solid, even while its fronds are buffeted by turbulence. Similarly, *hara* breathing enhances our capacity to claim and sustain inner ease because the breathing pattern works with our own physiology to settle the nervous system. By eliciting a shift from sympathetic to parasympathetic mode, *hara* breathing settles mind-body-emotions, anchoring us in the present moment, so we can relate intentionally to what is coming up in our inner lives and in the lives of others. When we practice *hara* breathing, we create a space of potential and possibilities; a spaciousness within which we access our inner strength and wisdom. We nourish and steady ourselves at that very moment in time.

The Mindful Pause (Ch. 4): When we practice a mindful Pause throughout our days, we become ever more mindful of our own emotional reactivity. We become aware that we have a choice in how we respond, and that we can respond more intentionally. With moment-to-moment mindfulness, we can pivot away from our knee-jerk conditioned reactions, and embody wisdom and compassionate speech and action toward self and others. With practice of the mindful Pause, we experience emotional freedom when we *choose* where to place our attention and energy, instead of being hijacked by the runaway train of the mind.

Joshin Kokyu-Ho (Ch. 5): When we practice *Joshin Kokyu-ho* meditation, our body and mind settle like the snow in a snow globe. With the refreshing in-breath, we stabilize the mind in the body. When we center the mind in this way, the less our thoughts wear us down or spiral us out of control. We cultivate a body and mind that is grounded and centered. With the expansive out-breath, we create openness, spaciousness, and emotional freedom. With the practice of *Joshin Kokyu-ho* meditation we sustain a pervasive sense of physical, mental-emotional, and spiritual well-being and ease.

Gassho **Meditation** (Ch. 5): The stillness and focus of *Gassho* meditation quiets the mind, and stillness is both an end in itself, and a means to larger ends. *Gassho* meditation invites us to notice each time our attention strays, and to return our awareness to the point where the middle fingers touch. This creates and sustains an inner terrain of mindfulness and composure that we carry with us so that our practice is reflected in our daily life.

Hands-On Self-Reiki Practice (Ch. 6): This embodied element of Reiki practice gets us in touch with the body in its physicality, deepening the mind-body connection, and bringing our attention to the present moment. When we experience this nourishing touch of the body, we are drawn into sustainable inner stillness, stability, and ease. As we feel into the contact between the hands and the body, we return control to the natural capacity of the body to heal. We can experience and appreciate the physiological benefits (Chapter 1) of hands-on self-Reiki practice.

3 Diamonds of *Ki* Meditation (Ch. 7): When we are mindful of our *body like a mountain, our mind like the sky, and our heart like the ocean*, we sense into our inner qualities of Earth *Ki* (body-stability), Sky *Ki* (mind-vast openness), and Heart *Ki* (heart-interconnection). With 3 Diamonds of *Ki* practice we become mindful of the state of our body, mind, and heart so we can live consciously aware and awake to all possibilities, while being grounded and settled. When we feel balance between Earth *Ki* and Sky *Ki*, we can express Heart *Ki* genuinely and naturally. We can live intentionally. From these three centers of awareness, we claim our courage to climb over, navigate around, or discover a way through, life's challenges, while remaining open and available to others.

All of the self-Reiki practices introduced in this book serve us in two interrelated ways: One way is to provide us with *in-the-moment* skills and practices with which to address the inevitable hardships in our lives and in the lives of others as they come up. The other way is to build and sustain our *ongoing* well-being – mind-body-spirit – even when things seem to be going fine. Among the most meaningful benefits of self-Reiki practice for both addressing hardships in the moment *and* sustaining enduring well-being are:

- quieting the mind
- steadying the body
- settling the emotions
- down-regulating the nervous system
- experiencing physiological benefits including reduction of pain, increased immune function, and decreased inflammation
- experiencing mindfulness
- bringing full awareness to our experiences
- increasing vitality and spirit
- becoming more familiar with ourselves and inviting insight into our habitual patterns
- fostering resilience and courage
- cultivating an inner spaciousness that opens us to possibilities
- creating the capacity to hold the unexpected without getting knocked down
- freeing ourselves to stretch beyond our own comfort zone
- opening the heart: overcoming separation and becoming conscious of connection – participatory consciousness
- nourishing ourselves and others with kindness and compassion
- cultivating a sacred outlook
- effecting change in the face of social injustice
- being at peace with self and others

Let's practice building this mind-body-spirit state together with a closing meditation to pave the way to walk in peace with self and others:

In this moment let's anchor ourselves.

- *Bringing attention inward to your breath.*
- *Breathing in, sensing the possibility of ease within yourself.*
- *Breathing out a slow, lengthened breath.*
- *Continuing your hara breathing.*
- *If it is comfortable, bringing your hands to a place on the body to which they are drawn.*
- *Like the snow in a snow globe, feeling your body settling.*
- *Like the snow in a snow globe, feeling your mind settling.*
- *Like the snow in a snow globe, feeling your emotions settling.*
- *Allowing yourself to soften.*
- *Sensing an expansive awareness of the potential for experiencing beauty in the everyday.*
- *Knowing we can walk together with purpose and on purpose in peace with self and others.*

In Gratitude

The system of Reiki teaches us to conclude each Reiki practice with an expression of gratitude to the practice itself, to our teachers, and to anyone who may be with us. We stand in deepest gratitude to our Reiki teachers and mentors, our Reiki colleagues, and all of those who placed their trust in us and in the practice of Reiki to cultivate wellness, mindfulness, and spiritual expression. We stand in utmost thanks and appreciation to our family and friends who offered loving encouragement during the book writing process. So, too, as we close this book, we state an intent of gratitude to you, the reader, for walking intentionally and peacefully with us. May your Reiki self-practice allow you to walk in peace with self and others.

References

Benson, Henry (1974) *The Relaxation Response*. NY: HarperCollins

Cassel, Eric (1982) The Nature of Suffering and the Goals of Medicine. *New England Journal of Medicine* 306(11):639-6345

Doi, Hiroshi (2014) *A Modern Reiki Method for Healing*, Revised Edition. Southfield, MI: Vision Publications

Doty, James MD (2017) *Into the Magic Shop: A Neurosurgeon's Quest to Discover the Mysteries of the Brain and the Secrets of the Heart*. NY: Avery, Penguin Random House

Ellyard, Lawrence (2006) *The Ultimate Reiki Guide for Beginners*. Washington: O-Books

Epstein, Ronald MD (2017) *Attending: Medicine, Mindfulness, and Humanity*. NY: Scribner

Felitti, Vincent J. MD, FACP A; Robert F. Anda MD, MS B; Dale Nordenberg MD C; David F. Williamson MS, PhD B; Alison M. Spitz MS, MPH B; Valerie Edwards BA B; Mary P. Koss PhD D; James S. Marks MD, MPH B (1998) Relationship of Childhood Abuse and Household Dysfunction to Many of the Leading Causes of Death in Adults. The Adverse Childhood Experiences (ACE) Study. *American Journal of Preventive Medicine*, May 1998, Volume 14, Issue 4, Pages 245-258

Field, Tiffany (2001) *Touch*. 2nd Edition. A Bradford Book. Cambridge: MIT Press

Fueston, Robert (2016) *The History and System of Usui Shiki Reiki Ryoho*. Lotus Press

Galea, Sandro (2019) *Well: What We Need to Talk About When We Talk About Health*. NY: Oxford

Harris, Nadine Burke MD (2018) *The Deepest Well: Healing the Long-Term Effects of Childhood Adversity*. Houghton Mifflin Harcourt Publishers

Jacobs, Barry (2018) Reframing the "Burden" of Caretaking: Why Accepting Help is Empowering for those Receiving and

Giving. *Psychotherapy Networker* newsletter, 5/3/2018

Jonas, Wayne (2018) *How Healing Works*. Lorena Jones Books, Ten Speed Press

Klagsbrun, Joan (2018) On Aging Courageously. *Psychotherapy Networker* newsletter, March 3, 2018

Langade, Deepak, et al. (2016) Burnout Syndrome Among Medical Practitioners Across India. *Cureus* 8 (9)

Leitch, Laurie: https://www.thresholdglobalworks.com/srm-a-strategy-for-uncertainity/

Lesser, Marc (2019) *Seven Practices of a Mindful Leader: Lessons from Google and a Zen Monastery Kitchen*. Novato, California: New World Library

Lewis, Katherine Reynolds (2018) *The Good News About Bad Behavior: Why Kids Are Less Disciplined Than Ever—And What to Do About It*. NY: Hachette

Magee, Rhonda (2015) How Mindfulness Can Defeat Racial Bias. *Greater Good Magazine*, University of California, Berkeley

McEwen, BS (1998) Stress, Adaptation and Disease. Allostasis and Allostatic Load. *Ann NY Acad Sci*. 1998: 840:33-44. [PubMed: 9629234]

Pearson, Nicholas (2018) *Foundations of Reiki Ryoho: A Manual of Shoden and Okuden*. Rochester, VT: Healing Arts Press

Petter, Frank Arjava (2012) *This is Reiki: Transformation of Body, Mind and Soul*. Wisconsin: Lotus Press, Shangri-La

Picard, et al. (2016) Mitochondrial functions modulate neuroendocrine, metabolic, inflammatory, and transcriptional responses to acute psychological stress. *Proceedings of the National Academy of Sciences of the United States of America*

Sapiro, Michael PsyD (2018) *The Self-Care Vow: Turning the Bodhisattva's Gaze Inward*

Shanafelt, Tait; Lotte Dyrbye; Colin West (2017) Addressing Physician Burnout: The Way Forward. *JAMA*. Published online, February 9, 2017

Siegel, Daniel and Tina Payne Bryson (2018) *The Yes Brain: How* to *Cultivate Courage, Curiosity, and Resilience in Your Child*. Bantam Books, Penguin Random House

Stiene, Bronwen and Frans –

(2005) *The Japanese Art of Reiki*. O-Books

(2008) Lessons from Usui Mikao Memorial Stone. *International House of Reiki*

Talbot, Simon G. and Wendy Dean (2018) Physicians aren't 'burning out.' They're suffering from moral injury. *Stat News*

Wilberg, Peter (2003) *Head, Heart & Hara: The Soul Centres of West and East*. London: New Gnosis Publications

Wilkinson, Richard & Kate Pickett (2011) *The Spirit Level: Why Greater Equality Makes Societies Stronger*. NY: Bloomsbury Press

Appendix

Reiki Research Papers, Compiled by Elise Brenner

Alandydy, Patricia BSN, RN (1999) Using Reiki to Support Surgical Patients. *Journal of Nursing Care Quality*, Vol. 13, No. 4, pp. 89-91.

Baldwin, AL and GE Schwartz (2006) Personal interaction with a Reiki Practitioner decreases noise-induced microvascular damage in an animal model. *Journal of Alternative and Complementary Medicine* 12(1):15-22.

Baldwin, AL; C. Wagers; GE Schwartz (2008) Reiki improves heart rate homeostasis in laboratory rats. *J. of Alt. and Comp. Med.* 14(4): 417-422.

Billot, Maxime; Maeva Daycard; Chantal Wood; Achille Tchalla (2019) Reiki therapy for pain, anxiety and quality of life. *BMJ Supportive and Palliative Care*, Volume 9, Issue 4.

Birocco, N.; Guillame, C.; Storto, S.; Ritorto, G.; Catino, C.; Gir, N.; Balestra, L.; Tealdi, G.; Orecchia, C.; Vito, GD; Giaretto, L.; Donadio, M.; Bertetto, O.; Schena, M.; Ciuffreda, L. (2012) The effects of Reiki therapy on pain and anxiety in patients attending a day oncology and infusion services unit. *Am J Hosp Palliat Care* 29(4):290-4.

Bowden, Deborah; Lorna Goddard; John Gruzelier (2011) Research Article: A Randomised Controlled Single-Blind Trial of the Efficacy of Reiki at Benefitting Mood and Well-Being. *Evidence-Based Complementary and Alternative Medicine*, Volume 2011, Article ID 381862, 8 pages.

Crawford, SE; VW Leaver; SD Mahoney (2006) Using Reiki to decrease memory and behavior problems in mild cognitive impairment and mild Alzheimer's Disease. *J. of Alt. and Comp. Med.* 12(9):911-913.

Cuneo, Charlotte; Maureen Curtis Cooper; Carolyn Drew;

Christine Naoum-Heffernan; Tricia Sherman; Kathleen Walz; Janice Weinberg (2011) The Effect of Reiki on Work-Related Stress of the Registered Nurse. *Journal of Holistic Nursing*, March 1, 2011.

Dyer, Natalie; Ann L. Baldwin; William L. Rand (2019) A Large-Scale Effectiveness Trial of Reiki for Physical and Psychological Health. *Journal of Alternative and Complementary Medicine*, December 2019: 1156-1162.

Fleisher, KA; Mackenzie, ER; Frankel, ES; Seluzicki, C.; Casarett, D.; Mao, JJ (2014) Integrative Reiki for cancer patients: a program evaluation. *Integrative Cancer Therapies* 13(1): pp. 62-67.

Foley, MK; Anderson, J.; Mallea, L.; Morrison, K.; Downey, M. (2016) Effects of Healing Touch on Postsurgical Adult Outpatients. *Journal of Holistic Nursing* 34(3): pp. 271-279.

Friedman, RS; Burg, MM; Miles, P.; Lee, F.; Lampert, R. (2010) Effects of Reiki on Autonomic Activity Early After Acute Coronary Syndrome. *J Am Coll Cardiol* 56(12):995-6.

Gantt, MeLisa AN, USA (Ret.); Judy Ann T. Orina CCRP (2019) Educate, Try, and Share: A Feasibility Study to Assess the Acceptance and Use of Reiki as an Adjunct Therapy for Chronic Pain in Military Health Care Facilities. *Military Medicine*, Volume 185, Issue 3-4, Pages 394-400.

Hammerschlag, Richard, et al. (2015) Biofield Physiology: A Framework for an Emerging Discipline. *Global Advances in Health and Medicine*, November 2015, Volume 4, Number suppl.

Henneghan, AM & Schnyer, RN (2015) Biofield Therapies for Symptom Management in Palliative and End-Of-Life Care. *American Journal of Hospice and Palliative Care* 32(1): pp. 90-100.

Jain, Shamini, et al. (2015) Clinical Studies of Biofield Therapies: Summary, Methodological Challenges and Recommendations. *Global Advances in Health and Medicine*, November 2015, Volume 4, Number suppl.

Jain, S.; McMahon, GF; Hasen, P.; Kozub, MP; Porter, V.; King, R.; Guarneri, EM (2012) Healing Touch with Guided Imagery for PTSD in Returning Active Duty Military: A Randomized Controlled Trial. *Military Medicine* 177(9): pp. 1015-1021.

Mackay, N.; Hansen, S.; McFarlane, O. (2005) Autonomic Nervous System Changes During Reiki Treatment: A Preliminary Study. *J. Altern Complement Med* 10 (6): 1077-1081.

Mansour, Ahlam; Marion Beuche; Gail Laing; Anne Leis; Judy Nurse (2007) A Study to Test the Effectiveness of Placebo Reiki Standardization Procedures Developed for a Planned Reiki Efficacy Study. *Journal of Alternative and Complementary Medicine*, September 2007 5(2).

McManus, David E. PhD (2017) Reiki Is Better Than Placebo and Has Broad Potential as a Complementary Health Therapy. *J Evid Based Complementary Altern Med* 22(4): 1051-1057.

Miles, P. (2007) Reiki for Mind, Body, and Spirit Support of Cancer Patients. *Advances in Mind-Body Medicine*, Fall 2007; 22(2):20-26.

Miles, P. (2003) Preliminary Report on the Use of Reiki for HIV-related Pain and Anxiety. *Alternative Therapies in Health and Medicine* 9(2):36.

Notte, BB; Fazzini, C.; Mooney, RA (2016) Reiki's Effect on Patients with Total Knee Arthroplasty: A Pilot Study. *Nursing* 46(2):17-23.

Pocotte, Susan L. PhD; Salvador, Diane MSN RN (2008) Reiki as a Rehabilitative Nursing Intervention for Pain Management: A Case Study. *Rehabilitation Nursing Journal* (2012).

Reese, Caroline (2019) Sensemaking and Identity in Complementary Alternative Medicine: Communication Study on Reiki. Master's Thesis, Marquette University.

Rosada, RM; Rubik, B.; Mainguy, B.; Plummer, J.; Mehl-Madrona, L. (2015) Reiki Reduces Burnout Among Community Mental Health Clinicians. *Journal of Alternative and Complementary Medicine* 21(8): pp. 489-495.

Rubik, Beverly, et al. (2015) Biofield Science and Healing: History, Terminology, and Concepts. *Global Advances in Health and Medicine*, November 2015, Volume 4, Number suppl.

Schmehr, R. (2003) Case Report: Enhancing the Treatment of HIV/AIDS with Reiki Training and Treatment. *Alternative Therapies in Health and Medicine* 9(2):120.

Shirani, Naser; Abdolghani Abdollahimohammad; Mohammad reza Firouzkouhi; Nosratollah Masinaeinezhad; Aziz Shahraki-Vahed (2019) The Effect of Reiki energy therapy on the severity of pain and quality of life in patients with rheumatoid arthritis: A Randomized clinical Trial Study. *Medical Science*, March-April 2019.

Thrane, Susan RN, MSN, OCN and Susan M. Cohen DSN, APRN, FAAN (2014) Effect of Reiki Therapy on Pain and Anxiety in Adults: An In-Depth Literature Review of Randomized Trials with Effect Size Calculations. *Pain Management Nursing* 15(4): 897-908.

Valdovinos, Rafael Rivera; Leticia Casique; Alicia Alvarez Aguirre (2019) Reiki as nursing care to increase self-esteem, improve family well-being and decrease the consumption of alcohol, tobacco and marijuana in young adults. *Hospice & Palliative Medicine International Journal* 3(2).

Vitale, Anne T. MSN, APRN, BC; O'Connor, Priscilla C. PhD, APRN, BC (2006) The Effect of Reiki on Pain and Anxiety in Women With Abdominal Hysterectomies: A Quasi-experimental Pilot Study. *Holistic Nursing Practice* 20(6): 263-272.

Vitale, Anne MSN, APRN, BC (2007) An Integrative Review of Reiki Touch Therapy Research. *Holistic Nursing Practice* 21(4): 167-179.

Webster, Lindsay; Janice Miner Holden; Dee C. Ray; Eric Price; Tessa M. Hastings (2019) The Impact of Psychotherapeutic Reiki on Anxiety. *Journal of Creativity in Mental Health*, DOI: 10.1080/15401383.2019.1688214.

Wong, J.; Ghiasuddin, A.; Kimata, C.; Patelesio, B.; Siu, A. (2013) The Impact of Healing Touch on Pediatric Oncology Patients. *Integrative Cancer Therapies* 12(1): 25-30.

Zins, Savannah PhD, RN; Mary Catherine Hooke PhD, APRN, PCNS, CPON; Cynthia R. Gross (2018) Reiki for Pain During Hemodialysis: A Feasibility and Instrument Evaluation Study. *Journal of Holistic Nursing* 37 (2):148-162.

Zucchetti, Giulia PhD; Filippo Candela PhD; Cristina Bottigelli RN, et al. (2019) The Power of Reiki: Feasibility and Efficacy of Reducing Pain in Children With Cancer Undergoing Hematopoietic Stem Cell Transplantation. *Journal of Pediatric Oncology Nursing* 36 (5):361-368.

BOOKS

SPIRITUALITY

O is a symbol of the world, of oneness and unity; this eye represents knowledge and insight. We publish titles on general spirituality and living a spiritual life. We aim to inform and help you on your own journey in this life.

If you have enjoyed this book, why not tell other readers by posting a review on your preferred book site?

Recent bestsellers from O-Books are:

The Heart of Tantric Sex
Diana Richardson
Revealing Eastern secrets of deep love and intimacy to Western couples.
Paperback: 978-1-90381-637-0 ebook: 978-1-84694-637-0

Crystal Prescriptions
The A-Z guide to over 1,200 symptoms and their healing crystals
Judy Hall
The first in the popular series of eight books, this handy little guide is packed as tight as a pill-bottle with crystal remedies for ailments.
Paperback: 978-1-90504-740-6 ebook: 978-1-84694-629-5

Take Me To Truth
Undoing the Ego
Nouk Sanchez, Tomas Vieira
The best-selling step-by-step book on shedding the Ego, using the teachings of *A Course In Miracles*.
Paperback: 978-1-84694-050-7 ebook: 978-1-84694-654-7

The 7 Myths about Love...Actually!
The Journey from your HEAD to the HEART of your SOUL
Mike George
Smashes all the myths about LOVE.
Paperback: 978-1-84694-288-4 ebook: 978-1-84694-682-0

The Holy Spirit's Interpretation of the New Testament
A Course in Understanding and Acceptance
Regina Dawn Akers
Following on from the strength of *A Course In Miracles*, NTI
teaches us how to experience the love and oneness of God.
Paperback: 978-1-84694-085-9 ebook: 978-1-78099-083-5

The Message of A Course In Miracles
A translation of the Text in plain language
Elizabeth A. Cronkhite
A translation of *A Course in Miracles* into plain, everyday
language for anyone seeking inner peace. The companion
volume, *Practicing A Course In Miracles*, offers practical lessons
and mentoring.
Paperback: 978-1-84694-319-5 ebook: 978-1-84694-642-4

Your Simple Path
Find Happiness in every step
Ian Tucker
A guide to helping us reconnect with what is really important in
our lives.
Paperback: 978-1-78279-349-6 ebook: 978-1-78279-348-9

365 Days of Wisdom
Daily Messages To Inspire You Through The Year
Dadi Janki
Daily messages which cool the mind, warm the heart and guide
you along your journey.
Paperback: 978-1-84694-863-3 ebook: 978-1-84694-864-0

Body of Wisdom
Women's Spiritual Power and How it Serves
Hilary Hart
Bringing together the dreams and experiences of women across
the world with today's most visionary spiritual teachers.
Paperback: 978-1-78099-696-7 ebook: 978-1-78099-695-0

Dying to Be Free
From Enforced Secrecy to Near Death to True Transformation
Hannah Robinson
After an unexpected accident and near-death experience, Hannah
Robinson found herself radically transforming her life, while a
remarkable new insight altered her relationship with her father, a
practising Catholic priest.
Paperback: 978-1-78535-254-6 ebook: 978-1-78535-255-3

The Ecology of the Soul
A Manual of Peace, Power and Personal Growth for Real People
in the Real World
Aidan Walker
Balance your own inner Ecology of the Soul to regain your
natural state of peace, power and wellbeing.
Paperback: 978-1-78279-850-7 ebook: 978-1-78279-849-1

On the Other Side of Love
A woman's unconventional journey towards wisdom
Muriel Maufroy
When life has lost all meaning, what do you do?
Paperback: 978-1-78535-281-2 ebook: 978-1-78535-282-9

Practicing A Course In Miracles
A translation of the Workbook in plain language, with mentor's
notes
Elizabeth A. Cronkhite
The practical second and third volumes of The Plain-Language
A Course In Miracles.
Paperback: 978-1-84694-403-1 ebook: 978-1-78099-072-9

Readers of ebooks can buy or view any of these bestsellers by
clicking on the live link in the title. Most titles are published
in paperback and as an ebook. Paperbacks are available in
traditional bookshops. Both print and ebook formats are
available online.

Find more titles and sign up to our readers' newsletter at
http://www.johnhuntpublishing.com/mind-body-spirit

Follow us on Facebook at https://www.facebook.com/OBooks/
and Twitter at https://twitter.com/obooks